Strength Training over 40

The Only Weight Training Workout Book You Will Need to Maintain or Build Your Strength, Muscle Mass, Energy, Overall Fitness and Stay Healthy Without Living in the Gym

Michael Smith

Strength Training over 40

Second Edition

By Michael Smith

Table of Contents

Introduction

"Never cease chiseling your own statue."
~ Plotinus

Did you know that once you cross the age of 40 you lose about one pound of muscle every year? I thought you should know. The adage, "use it or lose it," is specifically true when it comes to losing muscle as we age. A typical person starts experiencing a natural decline in muscle mass once they turn 30, and that loss speeds up as time passes. As a result, your body weakens and your muscles begin to lose strength, making you less flexible and more susceptible to injuries.

Most of us lead a technology-driven lifestyle. We no longer subject our bodies to the same workload our ancestors did. We use machines to do almost everything. As a result, our bodies have responded with a meltdown of muscle mass and strength since it is no longer in use. That's why people who remain physically inactive lose more muscle mass and strength as they grow older than those who stay physically active.

Research shows that muscle loss has detrimental effects on your body and overall health. It is associated with bone loss, joint and back pains, physical dysfunction, slow metabolism, and fat gain, just to mention a few.

As we grow older, most of us are worried that we are going to become frail, incapacitated, and incapable of taking care of ourselves. And we are silently wondering how we are going to fare in the last stages of our lives. We are generally hopeless about our overall well-being as the years pass. Don't despair. It's not too late. You can do something to offset Mother Nature. Yes, you can. I don't mean witchcraft, or anything related to black magic, but strength training.

A lot of medical and scientific studies have proven that strength training is the most important step you can take, not just to put a brake on muscle loss and slow down the aging process, but to reverse it and say goodbye to health-related problems that come with it. Before we dive deeper, let's understand what strength training is.

What is Strength Training?

Some people equate strength training to bodybuilding, but it is not necessarily the same thing. Strength training, also known as resistance training, is the use of your body weight, free weights (like dumbbells, barbells, kettlebells, etc.), or weight from gym machines to perform exercises designed to increase skeletal muscle strength and endurance. It requires that the muscles work against the weights and overcome them. You lift the weights in opposition to the downward force that gravity places upon them.

The goal of strength training, especially for individuals in their 40s and above, is to improve overall body strength, to become more potent physically, to maintain functional movement, and make daily activities more manageable. It also helps you stay fit and in good physical shape regardless of your age.

In addition, strength training builds muscles, though not at the same rate at which bodybuilding does. The term "bodybuilding" usually refers to competitive exhibitions, and a lot of "bodybuilders" are only working out to get the kind of body that will look good on a stage. This is a very challenging sport because it is not easy to balance bulking, cutting phases, and following a strict diet all the time.

Like any other professional sport, bodybuilding has little to do with health. I believe you now get the difference.

Whether you want to gain muscle or gain strength, you'll find that both goals require similar types of exercise - the difference lies in the number of reps you're doing, the weights, and rest time between sets. This will be explained in detail in chapter 5.

Common Strength Training Misconceptions Among Over 40s

Strength training is one of the most misunderstood aspects of exercise by people aged 40 and beyond. This is due to classic misconceptions that have been allowed to creep into our society regarding strength training and age. Most people above the age of 40 believe that:

- It is too late to start strength training
- They will hurt themselves as they exercise due to their age
- They can't move and lift weights like they used to in their 20s
- Walking or cardio is enough for them
- They have a weak heart and joints hence they can't withstand high intensity exercises
- Staying sedentary is the best way to prevent falls and injuries
- Exercise can lead to, or escalate, joint pain at this age
- Now that they have age-related health problems, exercise isn't safe for them
- They are too old to exercise

These misconceptions are the ones that hold back many people over 40 from enjoying the benefits of strength training. Although many people over 40 may be attracted to strength training by reports of improved bone health, increased independence and flexibility, reduced risk of osteoporosis, increased stamina, reduced depression, weight loss, etc., they are unable to exercise due to these misconceptions. This book dispels these misconceptions and provides you with facts about strength training over 40.

Aging doesn't have to mean a decline in health; it is only a decline in our abilities to adapt to change, disease, and injury. And that is something we have influence and control over. Strength training can provide the solution to this problem. Whether you've been a fitness nut for decades or are a novice to strength training, it is never too late to get in shape. Just use the strength training workout program in this book and you will build strength and muscles regardless of your age.

Some people fear that they have to spend considerable time lifting expensive weights or paying expensive gym membership fees. Let me make things clear, you don't need to exercise for hours daily to benefit from strength training.

As little as 30 minutes of proper strength training exercise a couple of times per week for about two or three months can reverse as much as 10-30 years of decline in strength and function. You also don't have to worry about buying expensive machines and equipment or subscription fees.

You can work out from anywhere without, or with minimal, gym equipment and still gain the same benefits as those who work out in gyms. Wondering how? Don't worry. Just read on. I will show you how to do it.

Studies indicate that exercise and proper diet are key factors in achieving good health and wellness, especially after 40. Research also predicts that millions of people across the globe will become weak as they age due to severe loss of muscle mass and strength. The greatest news is that you don't have to be among them.

There are actions you can take to help prevent the situation or reverse it. With over 20 years' experience in research on topics in the fitness, health, nutrition, and wellness field and knowing what I know about fitness, I must warn you that there are no special products for increasing muscle mass and strength or antiaging. Anyone who is trying to sell you such products is scamming you! To get a strong, good looking, and healthy body, you need to do strength training.

I have studied various fitness concepts while applying what I have learned to my own workout routine and my friends'. I have helped train hundreds of people in achieving their ideal body shape and stamina. Believe it or not, every single person I help achieve their fitness goals, from all ages, sizes, shapes, and abilities, I advise them to use strength training exercises, which work wonders. I get pleasure in motivating others and just having an overall passion for health and fitness.

I have tried all forms of workouts, including heavy weights, cardio-focused light weights, at-home workouts, organized classes, cycling, yoga, HIIT, total body, core strength, and dancing. This has enabled me to gain enough experience on matters concerning health and fitness. There is no secret formula to fitness success kept away from the public. It is simple, work out and eat healthy.

Before undertaking any exercise regimen, it is recommended that you consult your doctor. This is important as your doctor will be able to determine if your body is ready for exercise and advise you on the exercises you need to avoid depending on your health status.

Strength training is a beneficial activity. Just find your motivation, learn how to execute the exercises correctly and safely, be committed, stay consistent, take enough rest to allow your muscles to recover, and you will see the results.

So, if you're over 40 and looking for youthful, or want to build muscle mass, strength, flexibility, stay healthy and increase self-confidence, this book is meant for you. It has all the important information and guidelines that will help you do exactly that.

In the first chapter, I am going to show you why you can't afford to skip exercises, especially once we cross age 30, and what we need to do to get the most out of it. Let's dive in!

Chapter 1: Why You Can't Skip Exercise

"Just keeping yourself interested and motivated to train over a long period is often the biggest hurdle and one of the biggest factors for success in building sustainable muscle."

~ Craig Cecil

Strength training at any age has rewards, but it has more rewards after 40. Aging is inevitable. In fact, you should be happy that you can age; others may not have the opportunity. However, as you grow older, you undergo a natural progression that involves the natural loss of many things, including muscle mass and strength, which can put you at increased risks of chronic illnesses and reduced lifespan. And the only way to prevent this is to incorporate strength training.

In this chapter, I am going to show you how to find your fitness whys, discuss the easy ways you can boost your willpower and motivate yourself to exercise, and the benefits of strength training at 40 and beyond. Keep reading!

The Benefits of Strength Training Over 40

• **Maintain and rebuild muscle mass.** Most people begin to lose their muscle mass at the age of 30 and decline by 3-8 % each decade. When you hit 50, the decline increases to 5-10% (Briley, 2020). Therefore, getting into a regular strength training routine is a great idea. It helps maintain and rebuild the muscles. But if you don't do anything about it, you will end up losing more than half of your muscle mass by the time you're 80.

• **Increase flexibility, strength, and balance**. Strength training increases your strength, flexibility, and posture, which helps with balance and coordination while also lowering your chances of falling while you walk. Flexibility requires the coordination of several parts of the body, including muscles, bones, and joints. Balance, as we age, is crucial. Our balance is affected by other factors, including eyesight and inner ear problems. However, if we maintain our strength and range of motion, we will be less likely to lose our balance.

• **Promote healthy and strong bones.** Regular exercise helps maintain bone density and create healthy bones. As we age, our bones start losing their tissues. This puts us at increased risk of sustaining injuries and fractures because our bones become brittle and can easily break. Research has proved that people who exercise regularly, regardless of their age, develop strong bones, tissues, and muscles. When you put stress on your bones, they respond and adapt by growing more cells and becoming denser. Regular strength training will therefore help you build the bone tissues and slow the loss of bone density that comes with old age.

- **Improve brain health.** Several studies have proven that there is an association between muscle strength and cognitive functions in aging people. Greater muscle strength leads to better cognitive functions. When we say cognitive functions, we refer to brain functions relating to receiving, storing, processing, and using information. According to research by scientists at Florida Atlantic University, sarcopenia (a process by which people lose muscle mass and strength as they age) can heighten the risk of cognitive function impairment (Collins, 2020).

Strength training is good for your aging brain for so many reasons, including halting the progression of brain diseases like Alzheimer's, having neuroprotective properties, preventing memory loss, and creativity in the brain. Regular strength training will not only help you regain physical strength and rev up your metabolism, but it will also help you maintain a healthy brain.

- **Promote better sleep**. As you grow older, getting enough sleep becomes increasingly important for your general health and wellbeing. Studies show that people who exercise regularly have a healthier sleeping cycle. Regular exercise makes you fall asleep more quickly, have serene sleep at night, and wake up feeling more energized and refreshed.

- **Improve the lymphatic system of your body.** The lymphatic system is a series of nodes that disperses throughout your body to move lymph fluid. Lymph fluids help white blood cells fight off infections. So, the lymphatic system depends on body movement to circulate the lymphatic fluid all over the body. Therefore, as you move your muscles, you aid in pumping lymphatic fluid to all your body parts, creating proper circulation in the lymphatic system.

- **Enhance your mood.** Moving your body improves your mood. Also, it reduces feelings of anxiety and depression. Studies show that strength training helps individuals with emotional disorders. It also allows one to better cope up with stress. One study was conducted to test the impact of body movements in addressing anxiety. The participants who exercised several times a week projected better moods than those who did not exercise. Those who did not exercise at all exhibited negative moods. Therefore, exercising is important in preventing acute stress.

- **Improve your sex life**. Exercising helps in achieving a good sex life for both men and women. It increases the flow of blood that improves sexual function. Also, it helps to regulate psychosocial factors such as mood, stress, and confidence.

Easy Ways to Boost Willpower and Self-Control

Most of our unhealthy and bad habits are triggered by lack of willpower and self-control. And there is nothing that sabotages willpower and self-control like stress. If you are more stressed, you are likely to overeat, overspend, oversleep or not sleep enough, stay inactive both physically and socially, and do many other things that jeopardize your health and wellbeing.

Anything that causes stress drains our supply of willpower and reduces our self-control. It is through willpower and self-control that you will be able to exercise consistently and reap the most out of its many benefits.

Anything that reduces stress in our lives and improves mood improves our willpower and self-control. Here are some of the things you can do to reduce stress and boost your willpower and self-control:

• **Exercise Regularly.** Exercise is the best way to improve self-control in all aspects of our lives. For those looking for a "quick fix" for willpower, this is it. Research shows that regular exercise reduces stress, depression, anxiety, cravings for food and drugs, and improves our mood and brain function. And again, it doesn't take a lot to boost your willpower. In fact, studies show that as little as five minutes of low-intensity exercise is enough to reap these benefits. Any exercise you perform replenishes your willpower and energy, even if it seems too light. So, anytime you feel tired, demotivated, or short on time for exercise, just remember the bigger picture.

• **Get more rest.** If you don't get enough sleep, you are more likely to get stressed and fail to keep your good habits in play. Studies show that lack of sleep causes forgetfulness, impulsivity, poor planning, and hyperactivity, which are similar to the symptoms of ADHD.

• **Give or receive a massage.** Receiving a massage relieves stress. I don't need to cite any research to convince you of this. Studies also indicate that giving a massage has similar effects. This is according to research that was carried out by scientists at the University of Oxford and ORYGEN Research Centre (Mathews, 2021).

Other studies also show that massage reduces pain, anxiety, and depression. Make a deal with your better half to trade massages before bed and you will be surprised with the outcome. It doesn't take a lot to reap the many benefits of giving or receiving a massage. Just 10 or 15 minutes are good enough!

- **Change your perception of stress.** We all know that stress is associated with impaired mental and physical health and wellbeing, but what we fail to understand is that our perception impacts its effects. Getting more stressed about stress puts you in a mess.

A study conducted by scientists at the University of Denver found that if you can view the things that stress you differently, you can prevent yourself from causing greater damage to your body (Mathews, 2021). For example, you shouldn't make a frustrating situation an excuse for not working out. Instead, you can view it as an opportunity to practice a virtue like tolerance or patience. Tough and painful situations can also make you tougher.

- **Take a walk in a park.** If you read or listen to the stories of many successful innovators and history's greatest thinkers, you will notice that they valued long walks in nature. For instance, Tchaikovsky was so adamant about his twice-a-day walks because he felt they were very important for his health and creativity. Thomas Jefferson also took regular walks around his Monticello estate. Studies show that just taking 25 minutes to walk in a park can reduce frustration and improve mood (Mathews, 2021).

- **Make love move.** Stay more intimate. Increase the number of times you have sex in a week if you're not having much sex. Several studies have shown that regular sex reduces stress, anxiety, and depression and makes you happier, resilient, and boosts your mood.

- **Listen to classical music.** Research shows that classical music can engage you emotionally, sharpen your mind, lower blood pressure, reduce physical pain and depression, and make you get quality sleep. So, next time you feel stressed just put on some slow, quiet, soothing classical music.

- **Reduce the amount of time you spend on your phone, laptop, and television.** Studies have found out that staring at screens for a long time destroys your mind. The more time you spend on your computer and cellphone, the more you feel stressed. A study carried out by scientists at the University of Gothenburg found out that most symptoms related to poor mental health are associated with excessive use of technology (Mathews, 2021). People who use their computers and cellphones frequently without breaks increase their likelihood of getting stressed, sleep disorders, and depression.

- **Make use of aromatherapy.** You can reduce stress and promote relaxation by simply enjoying nice smells. Studies show that aromatherapy or rather the scent of certain essential oils like lavender, chamomile, geranium, etc., can help lower blood pressure, improve sleep quality, and reduce anxiety. Use a diffuser to incorporate it into a daily relaxation routine.

How to Find Your Fitness Whys

To be successful in your fitness journey, you need to have SMART goals. People who start strength training exercises with vague, unrealistic, uninspired, or irrelevant fitness goals tend to quit first. And they are easy to spot. They will always have excuses and reasons for falling off the wagon. They will always complain about how situations and circumstances have forced them to lead a sedentary and unhealthy lifestyle. If you want to succeed where masses fail, you must avoid these attitudes and behaviors. That's why in this section, we are going to do a little soul-searching.

1. What does your ideal body look like?

The main reason why most people exercise is the desire to achieve a certain body shape and strength. And I am sure that this is the major reason you are here. Every single person I know that is physically fit, including myself, is motivated by their physical appearance. I ,love and value my health but it would be a big lie if I told you that health was my number one reason for venturing into regular strength training.

Don't mistake me for a narcissist, though. There are plenty of fitness benefits, but I don't see anything wrong with playing a bit to our vanity if great looks make us more confident.

So, one of the ways to identify your fitness goal is by looking at your body now and visualizing how you want to look. Take a picture of the physical features you would like to have, and your desired body shape. Save these pictures on your phone, google drive, or somewhere that you can easily access. This action will make you feel like you're working towards achieving a real, desirable body shape.

2. What does your ideal body feel like?

This question enables you to explore the "hidden" benefits of staying physically fit. The more fit and in shape you are, the more your self-esteem, productivity, self-fulfillment, and self-confidence increase. Your mood and alertness improve, and you get to enjoy increased energy levels, clearer thinking, fewer aches, and higher quality sleep.

So, take a few minutes to imagine these feelings and write them in your journal. Write down what you would like to feel using positive statements. An example would be "I'm full of strength and energy," or "My self-esteem is always high."

3. Your Fitness Why Changes as You Change

Fitness can be an amazing journey if you stay on the path to success. As you exercise, you are probably going to experience some changes, not just in physical appearance, but also in willpower, confidence, health, strength, and motivation. As these changes occur, your fitness goals change too. You need to rewrite the new goals. Remember that your goals are part of the reason you made it this far, so don't forget about them. Instead, revisit your starting point and make brand new goals that will help you achieve the things you never thought possible.

Tracking Your Progress

You can only tell the direction you're headed if you can measure progress and express it in real numbers. The major reason why many people don't achieve their fitness goals is that they lack a consistent, objective way to measure their progress.

Much of your future success or failure is hinged on how well you track your progress. We have three elements of tracking progress: body composition, diet, and exercise. However, in this book, we are only going to need to track our body composition and exercise. Let's take a closer look.

Tracking Your Body Composition

Body composition tracking is vital for any fitness journey. It is important to understand that even when you do everything right, it may take longer than you expect to observe changes in your physical appearance. And this can make you lose hope and give up.

However, if you learn to track your body composition properly, you can avoid this problem; with correct body composition tracking, you can always know what is happening with your body, allowing you to make adjustments accordingly. Below are the steps to tracking your body composition:

1. **Weigh yourself daily then calculate weekly averages.** Due to fluid retention, glycogen levels, and bowel movements, your weight changes daily. It is normal to experience regular ups and downs. That's why it is important to weigh yourself every day and then calculate your weekly average. By doing so, you will be able to focus on the end results rather than getting too caught up in the daily fluctuations, which may cause unnecessary frustrations and confusion. If your average weight is increasing, you are gaining weight and if it is reducing, you're losing weight. Just as simple as that.

Here is the procedure:

- Weigh yourself naked, after using the bathroom, and before drinking or taking anything in the morning.
- After seven days, add up the daily weigh-ins and divide by seven to get the daily average weight.
- Record your averages on your notepad app, Google Sheet, or somewhere you can easily access.

2. **Take body measurements once per week.** Your weight alone cannot tell you how your body changes, even with excellent tracking. Weight tracking doesn't tell you what you're gaining or losing - is it muscles or fat? If you are a beginner to strength training and have fat to lose, expect to gain muscles and lose fat at the same time. This means that the numbers on your scale may not change as much as you expect. That's why it is important to record at least one body measurement every week. You may keep an eye on the circumference of your waist. Your waist size is a reliable indicator of fat loss or gain. Therefore, as you calculate your daily average body weight, measure the circumference of your waist at the end of every week and watch it over time.

Here is how to do it right

- Wrap a tape measure around your bare stomach, right at your navel

- Ensure that the tape measure isn't slanting and that it is parallel to the floor
- Snug your body slightly while ensuring that you don't compress the skin
- Breathe out as you take the measurements. Make sure that you don't flex or suck your belly in
- To ensure that your readings are consistent, measure in the same spot every time

3. **Take Progress Pictures Every Week.** Most of us are more concerned about what we see in the mirror than numbers. That's why some people prefer taking pictures rather than measurements. Therefore, it is significantly important to take your "before" pictures even if you don't like your appearance at that time. These pictures will make you love how your body transforms over the next few weeks and months. And you're probably going to be shocked at how much your physique has improved at some point. Make sure that you take weekly progress photos as you take your weekly measurements to see how the transformation unfolds.

Tracking your Exercise

Workout tracking is as important as body composition tracking. Tracking your strength training workout is the only way you can ensure that you are progressively overloading your muscles over time. Here are some of the methods you can use to track your exercise:

- **Keep a workout journal.** Journaling is one of the simplest and most effective ways to track your workout progress. By logging a workout journal, you can track the amount of weight you lift. This tells you whether you are getting stronger or not. Our bodies quite easily adapt to whatever exercises we consistently perform.

Therefore, if we keep lifting the same weights, performing the same reps, then our body can no longer elicit a response to change. This means that your muscles won't grow or get stronger. And this is the mistake that most of us make. This is where a workout journal comes in. It helps you put your muscles in a constant state of challenge.

- **Use a pen and paper.** This method of tracking exercise is as simple as it sounds. It is also the cheapest way of planning and tracking your workouts. All you need is a book and a pen; note down the exercises, the number of sets and reps you will be performing, the weights you will lift, etc.

- **Use your phone.** You can use any notes app or specific apps you like. I like to use google calendar to mark days for my strength workouts and days for other physical activities like going for a walk. The calendar helps me track my activity and to have enough rest between workouts. You can also add notes in calendar events for workouts if you need some help in tracking your weights and number of reps, but I don't use this. I'm content with having a picture of my workout on my phone to check if I missed any exercise.

Getting Motivated to Exercise

We have several ingredients that spice up a consistent exercise program - knowing exercise whys and setting smart goals, being prepared, discipline, commitment, etc. But there is one which is most important and sometimes most elusive - motivation. Your mentality is an important part of your long term muscle and strength building program. Of course, you need the weights, the reps, the sets, and the rest to develop lean muscle mass, but your state of mind will determine whether you start and stay consistent.

Several things may lower your motivation to exercise, especially if you have to do it from home. But the good news is that there are several ways to address barriers to exercise and get motivated. Here are a few of the options you can consider:

● **Set goals**. Before you get started with your strength training program, take some time to define your goals. Set a few realistic short-term and long-term goals that account for your circumstances and priorities. Identify what you want to achieve and how you need to carry out your plan.

- **Prepare for the exercise.** Know the workout you will do, the time it will take you, and what you will need to do it. Ensure that you have everything you need for every exercise.

- **Start slowly.** Don't jump into a high-intensity exercise program if you haven't been exercising. Start small and work your way up. You can start by spacing your workouts in 10-minutes increments twice a day with as little as 3 reps of 2 sets in each exercise. If you have ongoing heart problems or fear falling, start with easy chair exercises. This will help you slowly increase your fitness and confidence.

- **Reward yourself for exercising**. For every workout you do, no matter how small it is, don't forget to reward yourself. For example, if you exercised for 30 minutes in the morning, you could spend an hour listening to your favorite music, watching your favorite movie, or reading a novel. You can also plan for a bigger reward like a safari. Knowing that you will get a treat after working out is a great motivator.

- **Keep track of your exercise progress.** Measuring and celebrating your achievements is the best way to stay motivated to work out. To achieve this, track your daily exercises, measure your weekly and monthly progress to see if you've improved, and then update your exercise plan based on your progress.

- **Find ways to make it enjoyable.** Be creative. Find something that will help you stay consistent with your workout routine. Remember, strength training is not something that people love, but you can find something good about it. You may even start by lifting your children as you play with them, walking your dog, etc. Just do something that you enjoy, but remember to keep up the pace.

- **Make exercise a social activity.** If you want to succeed in your fitness goal, consider exercising with other people. Activities are always more enjoyable when done with others. Exercising alone can get you demotivated and make it easy to give up. If possible, get a workout buddy or an accountability partner. You may try a dance class, use family gatherings to do outdoor activities, join a charity run, or play team sports with your children.

Strength training gets easier once you get going. Developing a habit of working out regularly plays a bigger role in achieving your fitness goals and reaping the benefits of strength training even at an older age.

Motivation is one of our greatest struggles in this journey. However, it is important to think about what you are going to gain from exercising rather than just letting your motivation fade away. People who work out, including me, make every effort to look for reasons to do it. They know that exercise makes life better. So, if you find that you're not motivated to exercise, just think about its benefits.

Key Takeaways

- Strength training is beneficial at any age, but it is even more beneficial at age 40 and above.

- It is through willpower and self-control that you will be able to exercise consistently and get the most out of it.

- If you want to benefit from exercise and reach your full potential in health and fitness, you must be mentally motivated and prepared for the journey ahead.

- People who start strength training exercises with vague, unrealistic, uninspired, and irrelevant fitness goals always quit first. Don't be among them. Find 'smart' fitness whys.

Chapter 2: Maximizing Fitness Gains: Strength Training vs. Cardio Workouts

"Get off the treadmill of consumption, replication, and mediocrity. Begin lifting the weights of creativity, originality, and success."
~ Ryan Lilly

Have you been running several times a week and not getting results? You may wonder why these workouts do not seem to work. I have witnessed many disappointed people who practiced cardio for many hours without witnessing any physical changes. I would hate for you to go through the same.

Don't get me wrong, regular cardio exercises, such as running, cycling, and swimming, strengthen the heart muscles, increase lung capacity, burn calories, and may help to manage body weight.

Ideally, a balanced fitness regimen often includes a combination of both cardiovascular exercise and strength training. World Health Organization guidelines and recommendations highlight how much and what kind of physical activity adults need for good health:

- at least 150–300 minutes of moderate-intensity aerobic physical activity

- or at least 75–150 minutes of vigorous-intensity aerobic physical activity; or an equivalent combination of moderate- and vigorous-intensity activity throughout the week
- muscle-strengthening activities at moderate or greater intensity that involve all major muscle groups on 2 or more days a week

In essence, you should ideally do at least five 30-minute cardio workouts and at least two strength training workouts a week.

But if don't think that you could stick to seven workouts per week and want to get the results you want with the least amount of effort - the secret to losing your body fat and gaining muscle is through strength training. And the best part is that you can achieve your goals with only two to three strength training workouts per week.

During strength training, metabolism drives the lean muscle tissue to burn calories during the workout and the rest of your day. Unbelievable, right? Strength training improves your posture and physique. Additionally, it improves your cardio and helps you carry out other activities more efficiently as you burn calories.

Although most people prefer cardio exercises such as jogging, swimming, or biking, a lot of studies indicate that it is not the most effective in losing weight and building muscles. Studies show that some people even end up heavier than they started when they only focus on cardiovascular exercises. Cardio does not always guarantee significant results. Typically, replacing the burned calories is very easy.

For instance, if a person runs vigorously for 30 minutes, he is likely to burn approximately 300 calories (only up to 200 calories when doing low-impact cardio). Surprisingly, the same number of calories could be replaced by consuming a piece of bagel, donut, burger, or a couple of cans of cola. So, which is easier? Hitting the treadmill for half an hour or skipping the bagel? Furthermore, with or without exercise, our bodies burn about 100 calories every hour and you should deduct that from the "calories burned" that you see on the treadmill's screen.

It is more important to be conscious about your nutrition as you exercise. Have proper nutrition habits that back up your workout plan.

Apart from burning fewer calories than required, cardio makes your body adapt to calorie-reduction exercises. Scientists state that when your body is in a calorie deficit, the efficiency of energy production reduces, and as you work out, the energy required to perform the same exercises decreases. As a result, you do not burn as many calories as you may think as you perform the same exercises you started with under the same conditions. In such a case, you likely overeat, which stalls weight loss efforts. The only solution when this happens is increasing your cardio intensity to make up for the energy lost. However, it may lead to muscle loss and reduction of body metabolic rate. So evidently, cardiovascular exercises may not be the way to achieve the body you want.

If you're like most guys, you want to be strong, muscular, and athletic. Most often this is the reason why we start to exercise with weights. Cardio can't offer you the same results. Take athletes or people who run a lot but don't strength train, most of them are always skinny without noticeable muscles and you may also find that some have skinny-fat body composition. But now, look at those people who never run but perform weightlifting exercises consistently; most of them have well-defined muscle mass, buffed chest and arms, and strong big bodies. So, what kind of body do you prefer? The choice is yours.

If you're like most women, you want a toned body that is well sculptured. To be honest, cardio can never give you such body shape. You will need to perform strength training exercises. However, due to a common misconception that weightlifting makes you bulky, most women tend to avoid it. But the fact is that the low testosterone levels is one of the main reasons that women won't get bulky from lifting weights. Testosterone is a natural anabolic steroid, which directly stimulates muscle growth. And, on average, women only have one-seventh the amount of testosterone as men. In case you've seen any bulky woman, odds are they use steroids.

So why do I insist on strength training?

You don't need to lift weights all day to gain results from strength training; you can achieve significant results by strength training for 30 minutes a couple of times a week. As you consistently strength train, your muscles improve. After every exercise, you can gain strength to lift more weight.

As you exercise, your body adapts to burning excess fats. Strength training speeds up your body's metabolic rate which allows you to break down calories for an extended period after working out. Several studies have shown that in every 3 pounds of lean muscle, your body loses about 129 calories per day.

Strength training challenges your muscles to become stronger, giving you desirable results quickly. Through this, your body image improves, improving self-confidence. Lifting weights strengthens muscles by creating resistance. The tissues break down quickly, which triggers the body to heal the tissue. In this process, the muscles grow as they become stronger. Therefore, you should push your muscles to the point of fatigue regularly; however, as a beginner, start with a simple basic plan and level up with time.

Strength training strengthens the area around the joints, unlike cardio which strains the joints. Once your joints are strong, your range of movement and ability to perform additional weightlifting movements increases. If you practice weightlifting properly, the core areas of our joints increase the flow of your movement. Therefore, as you carry out the training, your body learns how to tolerate these movements, which reduces the risk of injury during the workout.

You may practice strength training at home or in the gym. Some of the common choices of strength training include:

- **Body weight.** This may be practiced with little to no equipment. Examples include pushups, pullups, planks, lunges, and squats.

- **Resistance bands.** This is an inexpensive method of using lightweight bands to create resistance. There are many types of resistance bands sold in sporting goods stores.

- **Free weights.** This strength training method involves classic training tools. Kettlebells and dumbbells are great choices to consider. If you have no access to free weights in your home, you use a gallon of water or sand; you may also improvise the car spare parts that you no longer use.

- **Weight machines.** They are offered in fitness centers. You can as well purchase one to use at home.

- **Suspension training.** This involves suspending part of your body. For instance, you may suspend your legs while performing push-ups or planks.

Overall, it is beneficial to move your body rather than staying inactive. If you get frustrated by the thought of exercising daily, then at least try to move your body. Don't just be a couch potato. Even just walking for ten minutes can make a difference. I want you to drop the belief that you need to cover miles to be considered an exercise. Starting with your brain to your joints, making simple and small movements can improve your health and create a significant impact in attaining a physically fit body.

Therefore, I advise you to move and avoid remaining inactive. Look for any activity that you love doing and make a commitment to indulge every day. For instance, if you love taking a walk, remind yourself to walk 30 minutes daily. Whether walking, swimming, golf, or any other low-intensity sports, have the discipline to practice it consistently and you will achieve good results.

Research shows that one of the major reasons why human beings have a brain is to produce adaptable and complex movements. It is through movements that we perform our daily activities. The most important aspect for to understand that body movement helps in maintaining good health. Many people have adopted a negative attitude towards the word exercise. They associate it with stress and obligation. By reading this book, you now understand that strength training has a positive impact on your health—see exercising as simply moving. You should never make it seem too difficult.

So, if working out is a negative vibe for you, try changing your mentality. Meanwhile, you must ensure that you stay physically active by moving your body. One of the simplest ways you can do this is walking around while talking to someone on the phone, especially when the call is with someone you talk to a lot. You may also just walk around your house as you pick up dirt or misplaced items or visit the nearest park for a stroll. All such movements add up. They have a tremendous significant effect on both your physical and mental health. The good thing is that you can try them in the comfort of your home without even having to change into your gym clothes. Some of the other ways you can move your body include:

● Decluttering and tidying your garage or basement. As you do this, you will be lifting some heavy items from one place to another, bending, squatting to pick stuff up, etc.
● Going shopping on foot.
● Shoveling snow during winter.
● Swimming in a lake or river during summer.
● Gardening is also another good exercise. It involves walking, squatting, moving your hands, pushing, and pulling. All these are healthy ways to move your body.
● Enjoy the outdoors. You may walk your dog, ride a bike, go hiking, or jog. As you move your body outside your house, you expose yourself to nature, improving your mental health.

Moving your body is generally healthy. So, if working out sounds like a burden to you, then do some simple movements that incorporate motion in your daily life and make you feel good. Based on what you like, you may switch your exercise training to fit your preferences. Without sacrificing your enjoyment, you can reach your exerting goals much more effortlessly.

To keep your body moving, balanced, strong, healthy, and in good shape, you need strength training as it helps burn more fat while preserving your muscles within a short time, unlike cardio. Now that we know this, let's find out what you will need for your strength training exercise.

Key Takeaways

- You don't need any cardio to get the strong, healthy, and good-looking body that you want, but you need strength training.

- Women can never bulk up no matter the amount of weight they lift. Their hormones do not favor that. But for men, yes! Their hormones allow it.

- Moving your body is healthy. Don't just be a couch potato. If you can't strength train right away, start by making simple movements.

- It is more important to be conscious of your nutrition than focusing on cardio exercises.

Chapter 3: You Will Need A lot of Exercise Equipment, Won't You?

"The road to nowhere is paved with excuses."
~ Mark Bell

By now, you know why it is important to strength train as you approach middle-age and even after. I can't stress enough that strength training is the best way to get in shape and build body strength. The question is whether you need a lot of equipment to perform the exercises. And if you need them, what should you go for?

If you are like me who has been using strength training exercises to keep fit, then you will agree that you need minimal equipment to perform most exercises. And if you are new to strength training, forget all the rumors you've heard. Strength training does not require fancy or expensive weightlifting equipment or gym-style machines.

You can even improvise using furniture or an item in your house and use it to do the exercises if your budget is tight. However, it is worthwhile to invest in at least one or two pieces of equipment to get the most out of your exercise routine. And free weights are a great choice!

You can use bodyweight exercises too, but even with such workouts, you will need some equipment like pull-up bars and parallel bars which can be complicated to install and use at home. But free weights are simple and easier to handle. That's why I believe they are the best option for anybody interested in weightlifting.

Free weights are weight training equipment like dumbbells, kettlebells, weight plates, weight sets, etc. Using free weights is an excellent way to lose extra fat and gain more strength and muscle. What makes free weights effective and efficient fitness tools for strength and muscle building is their ability to fully engage all the muscles in the body.

If you are serious about shaping up and building body strength, you need to get yourself a kettlebell or dumbbell. Here are some of the advantages of free weights:

- **They are functional.** Good exercise should improve your performance outside the gym. This is what we refer to as functional fitness or cxcrcisc. Free weights allow for a more natural motion that conforms to your body's functional movement, unlike machines which restrict the body to a single plane of motion. Even a basic free weight exercise like standing dumbbell biceps curl uses the hands as you would in your daily activities such as lifting grocery or shopping bags. As you get older, it is especially important to maintain this natural full functionality of movement.

• **They make you stronger.** How your body reacts to free weights is different from the response to machines. For example, free weight squatting and machine squatting have different impacts on your muscles. Squatting with free weight activates your muscles more with greater hormonal response. The hormones help your muscles to grow and rebuild as you train (Fetters, 2019).

• **They are portable.** Can you pack resistance machines in your traveling bag? Or fit them in your closet? Probably not. But a piece of lightweight dumbbell? That's totally possible. So, if you want to save serious cash and space, consider investing in free weights.

• **They improve your balance.** Unlike machines which restrict the weight movement in one plane of motion, free weights force your muscles to balance the weight in all planes. This makes your muscles work together, which helps improve balance, coordination, and better muscle growth.

• **They are more versatile.** Free weights are not limited to any specific exercise. With a set of kettlebells or dumbbells and a few square feet of space, you can perform a variety of exercises that work your muscles in different ways to strengthen them. Besides promoting muscle growth, varied exercise can make your workouts more interesting, motivating you to stay consistent with your regimen.

- **Free weights are more efficient.** Unlike machines which are fixed to a certain path forcing you to push or pull in one direction, free weights incorporate the stabilizing muscles that enable you to perform the movement. You also have to balance the weights and your body. This makes free weights more effective in producing overall muscular strength and power gains.

- **They reduce your risk of injury.** Lifting free weights shore up your muscle imbalances thus preventing injuries. Since free weights challenge your balance constantly during exercise, they force you to work and strengthen your stabilizing muscles, creating stability to help support your body and joints. You can get dumbbells and kettlebells of different weights, giving you a chance to adjust the weights to what you can lift comfortably and safely.

- **They burn more calories.** Free weights not only improve your stability, but also ensure that your entire body performs compound movements. When you work out more muscles, you burn more calories. For instance, if you perform kettlebell goblet squats, you work your legs, core, arms, and shoulders, increasing the number of calories burned compared to if you were performing an exercise that isolates a single muscle like calf raises.

- **They are less expensive.** Free weights are affordable. If you are serious about attaining a strong, good-looking, and healthy body, you can afford at least a dumbbell or kettlebell. A little money spent is worth the gain.

Strength training using gym machines can be intimidating. So, when it comes to developing a healthy and safe strength training program, free weights are the smarter route to take.

Let's have a closer look at some of the most common, efficient, and effective free weights used in strength training—kettlebells and dumbbells.

The Kettlebell

A kettlebell is a cast-iron ball with a handle on the top. Kettlebells come in different weights and can help burn up to 400 calories in 20 minutes (Smith, 2020). A kettlebell can be used to perform exercises like squats, lunges, shoulder presses, hinges, and lifts. As you work out with a kettlebell, your heart pumps a bit faster, burning almost 20 calories per minute.

Kettlebell enhances flexibility as you can use different moves in your workout. Kettlebell workouts usually are characterized by high-paced cardio and strength training moves. The key areas that it targets are the core, arms, legs, shoulders, and back.

The Dumbbell

Dumbbells are short bars with weights on the end, which can be fixed or adjustable to provide a variety of weights. All you do is adjust the setting to match your needs. For a household with more than one person needing to work out, adjustable dumbbells are the best.

Dumbbells are also great for isolation exercises. If your goal is working specific muscles like biceps, bicep curls using a dumbbell is the best choice.

Advantages of Kettlebells/Dumbbells

• They require little space for storage. You can use them to work out and store them in the corner of the room and use the area for other activities.
• They are multipurpose.
• They are inexpensive compared to other gym equipment.
• They promote coordination and stability of muscles and joints.

- They increase the flexibility of your muscles and joints, helping you attain functional strength.
- They improve your cardiovascular endurance.
- Kettlebell workouts can burn up to 20 calories per minute.
- They help improve body and mind coordination.
- Most dumbbells are adjustable, giving you a chance to gradually increase the amount of weight you're lifting. This enables you to build your muscles the proper way.

What you should know about these free weights

- Kettlebells, as well as dumbbells, cost around $10 to $100, depending on the weight. The heavier the kettlebell, the more expensive it is.
- It is advisable to sign up for a class to understand the basics kettlebell/dumbbell workouts, especially if you are a beginner.

- Kettlebells/dumbbell workouts can be done indoors or outdoors. You can also decide to join a gym class with a kettlebell/dumbbell workout.

Which is better, kettlebell or dumbbell?

None of them is distinctly superior to the other. You can use a kettlebell to perform any exercise as you would use a dumbbell. But I prefer kettlebells because they add more excitement to my workouts.

So, do you wish to pump your workout? Kettlebells are the way to go. They help burn more calories within a short time. Depending on the program, a kettlebell workout may involve both strength training and cardio exercises. Therefore, it is good to consult a health expert before you begin. Achieving desirable results using a kettlebell workout starts with your state of mind.

Adopt a ready mindset and ensure that you treat the workout with respect. By this, I mean that you have to be disciplined enough not to skip any workout.

Additionally, it is good to evaluate what works best for you. Some kettlebells may be too heavy for you, which may cause injuries to the shoulders, back, or neck. Therefore, ensure you are fully informed on how to use kettlebells by an experienced trainer who will guide you to avoid any risk of injury during the exercise. If you have been exercising before, using a kettlebell will be a great way to burn more calories in less time. Also, your muscles and stamina will build much faster.

The good thing about kettlebells is that you can use them for both high and low intensity exercises. I am going to use the kettlebell to explain how to perform the exercises in our program. However, this doesn't mean that you must perform the exercises using a kettlebell. If you have a dumbbell or prefer any other free weight, you are free to use it.

What if you have a health condition? Can you use free weights?

In such a case, a doctor's recommendation is necessary. Therefore, if your doctor approves, you can use free weights in your fitness routine. Using free weights in your workouts can also help reduce blood pressure and cholesterol levels. However, if you have any heart disease, checking with your doctor first should be the first step before adopting any free weight exercise.

Since it is a high-impact program, kettlebells exert pressure on your hip, back, shoulder, knees, and neck muscles. So, in case you have conditions, such as arthritis, that cause pain in your knees or back, you should go for less risky strength training programs like using body weight. Because of this, I have also included alternative exercises you can perform without equipment.

In case of any other health conditions, seek the guidance of an experienced instructor to assess the workout program that is appropriate for you.

To get the most out of free weight workouts, you must learn the techniques of exerting force as you lift them.

When you practice using the proper form, it is easier to avoid injuries.

I am going to discuss this in the next chapter. We will be learning how to lift free weights in the correct form. We are also going to include a bodyweight option for all core exercises. However, I believe that the most effective option for doing core movements is with weights, especially kettlebells. The greatest thing about using free weights is that you can use them to exercise anywhere, including outdoors, gyms, in your house, etc.

Key Takeaways

● You don't need a lot of equipment for strength training exercises. A kettlebell or dumbbells will help you perform most of the strength training exercises and reap the benefits.

● Just a single kettlebell can fully engage all muscles in the body.

● Free weights like kettlebells and dumbbells are affordable and adjustable. You can get one from $10 to $100. You can also have different weights as you progress to lifting heavier weights.

Chapter 4: Master the Moves

"You do not need to do many different exercises to get strong - you need to get strong on a very few important exercises, movements that train the whole body as a system, not as a collection of separate body parts. The problem with the programs advocated by all the national exercise organizations is that they fail to recognize this basic principle: the body best adapts *as a whole organism* to stress applied to the whole organism. The more stress that can be applied to *as much of the body at one time* as possible, the more effective and productive the adaptation will be."

~ Mark Rippetoe

In this chapter, I will introduce the six best compound exercises to increase overall muscle mass, strength, and achieve your desired body shape. A compound exercise involves multiple joints and training many muscles at once, allowing you to lift heavier weights and raise growth hormone and testosterone levels. This means time efficiency, faster muscle growth, and other benefits.

When describing each move, I will introduce and focus on my recommended exercise and afterward, alternative variations. Each exercise included here meets the expectations of the program. I did thorough research to ensure that I am providing you with a group of exercises that will work together to provide maximum results without extensive effort.

These exercises are meant to make you better, not worse. And to achieve this, you need to execute them correctly. So, start slow, follow all the instructions keenly and see the results! Let's get started!

1. Squats

Squats are the best exercise for leg development and possibly the best overall exercise to perform if you want to strengthen your body. This exercise is known as the king of all exercises. Squatting is something we were born to do and everyone across the world has done it. It is one of the first movements during childhood.

Babies begin with squats before they start walking upright. Unfortunately, once we grow up, we no longer embrace it.

Most people think about the barbell back squat when we mention squat as an exercise. Although this is the most famous variation of the squat, it is not the only one, nor is it the variation I recommend. Barbell back squats require a lot of energy, a trainer (if you're new to it), a squat rack, and a barbell with weights. You can't have all these at home. That's why I am recommending simple variations that you can perform anywhere, such as the goblet kettlebell squat.

The goblet kettlebell squat

This is one of the most effective squat variations you can do. It is also among the simplest full-body exercises to perform. It works your quads, glutes, calves, and core. And since you engage your hands by holding the weight, it also works your biceps, improving your arm and grip strength.

Its advantages

- It doesn't compromise the range of motion or form to achieve stability like other heavier squat variations.
- Holding a kettlebell at your chest provides a counterbalance which helps improve and reinforce a good posture and alignment during the movement, making it simpler and easier to perform the goblet squat safely and correctly.

- It has a shorter learning curve, hence an excellent teaching tool for learning how to perform classic squat variations correctly.

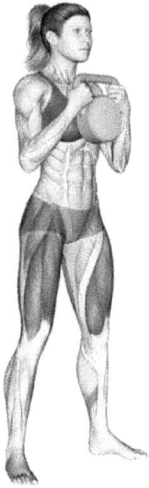

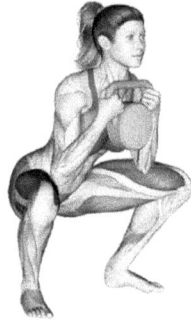

Instructions:

• Start by standing upright, holding a kettlebell in front of your chest with both hands by the sides of its handle. Your shoulders should be drawn back and downward and your elbows tucked in so that they are closer to the kettlebell. Keep your forearms as vertical as you can. Your feet should be just a tad wider than your shoulders.

• Take a deep breath in and brace your core. Keep your chest up and your back straight, hinge at the hip, and sit back as if you are sitting down on an invisible chair. Continue lowering yourself down as far as you can while keeping your head and chest up and your back straight.

- As you descend, push your knees apart. You should be able to feel most of your weight spread between your heel and midfoot.

- Don't round your lower back. Stop and come back up if you feel your lower back beginning to round. Don't lean forward or struggle to hold the bell upright. Your torso should remain vertical.

- Don't bend or twist your torso.

- Exhale as you stand back up. Put equal weight on both legs, ensuring your heels remain planted on the floor. Your knees, hip, and back should move at the same speed to ensure you maintain an upright posture throughout the entire movement.

Common form mistakes to avoid

- **Leaning forward.** Like any other squat variation, the kettlebell goblet squat requires you to keep your chest up every time you are performing this move. This helps keep your center of gravity on your feet.

- **Leaning back.** This helps keep your lats tight during the entire movement, enabling your body to stay balanced and stable. To achieve this, imagine someone is trying to tickle you from behind and draw your elbows in towards your sides.

- **Wobbling.** Ensure that you start each rep with your entire torso fully engaged. This helps keep you more stable, creating a smoother and controlled movement. Focus on tightening and tensing your lower back, abs, and glutes.

Alternatively, you can do this move with a dumbbell or resistance band. And if you are a novice or have physical limitations that might impair this movement, try bodyweight squats or bodyweight squats using TRX belt, chair or box squats, or even shallow knee bends.

2. The Hinge

The hinge is one of the most effective and efficient exercises for overall health and wellbeing. Unfortunately, it is the most neglected. Most of us spend a lot of time sitting, straining the back and spine, causing back pains. Also, as we grow older, most people tend to complain of back and joint pains. Luckily, these pains can be treated. And the best treatment option is to practice hinge exercises. Here are some simple exercises that incorporate the hinge:

The kettlebell swing

I believe that the kettlebell swing is the best option for hinge exercises! Pavel Tsatsouline, the founder of kettlebell training in the US and author of several books, noticed that kettlebell swing has many benefits, including improvement in the number of reps you can perform in a pull-up exercise and strength improvement in others.

Pavel, in one of his books, presents a minimalistic workout that consists of only 2 exercises: swing being one of them. This tells you how effective this exercise is. The kettlebell swing is not just a full-body exercise, it is what most experts refer to as a full-body response exercise. It has so many benefits on your muscles and the entire body. To get started and reap the most out of this exercise, here is how to go about it.

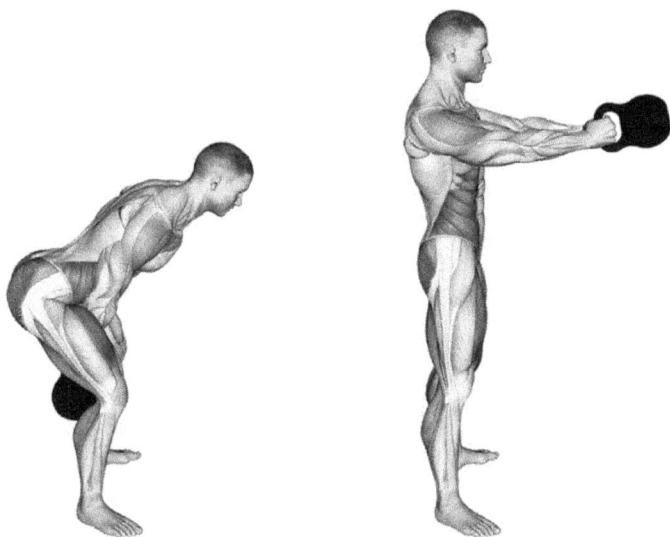

Instructions:

- Place a kettlebell on the ground right in front of your feet.

- Stand upright with your feet slightly wider than shoulder-width apart with the toes pointed slightly outward. Bend your knees slightly, roll back your shoulders and pull in your navel to engage your abs.

- Push your hips back and tip your torso forward to reach the handle of the kettlebell. As you do this, ensure that your back is completely straight and that you're not squatting.

- Breathe in as you comfortably grasp the handle of the kettlebell with both hands, your shoulders back. This helps control the momentum of the swing. Remember to keep your core engaged throughout the exercise.

- To begin the swing, hike the kettlebell back between your legs such that the kettlebell is extended behind your back. Exhale as you rise to an upright position. Don't extend your hips past your shoulders. Also, let the bell swing forward as high as it can naturally go.

- Breathe in and swing the kettlebell back to the floor through your legs in a slow and controlled motion, then exhale and repeat.

Common Form Mistakes to Avoid

- **Squatting as you swing.** Remember, kettle swing is a hinge movement, not a squat. This means that instead of bending at the knee, you should press your hips back any time you make the downward swing. The shins should stay mostly vertical.

- **Rounding your back.** A rounded or slumped shoulders and upper body indicate that your core and shoulder stabilizers are not properly engaged and could cause lower back pain or strain. To avoid this, try as much as possible to keep your spine and back straight.

- **Lifting with arms and shoulders.** Most people engage their shoulders and arms in the forward movement of the kettlebell. The hips should be moving the kettlebell, not your arms. Your arms should just hold the kettlebell, not raise it. Keep your shoulders and upper back in a relaxed but stable position. Try as much as possible to rely fully on the momentum of your hip extension to swing the weight.

Alternative hinge exercises

If you are a newbie or have physical limitations that might impair this move, try more simplified hinge variations like kettlebell deadlift or bodyweight alternatives like hip raise and standing back extensions.

The kettlebell deadlift

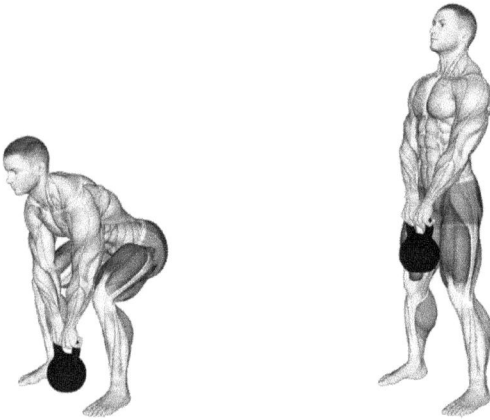

Instructions:

- Stand upright with a kettlebell between your feet.

- Push your hips backward while keeping your back straight.

- Bend your knees while maintaining a straight back with your chest lifted, and grab onto the handles of the kettlebell with both hands.

- Push into the ground to stand up. While keeping your arms straight, lift the kettlebell just above your knees. Ensure that your glutes are tight and you're not leaning backward.

- This counts as one rep.

Precautions to take

- To avoid injuries, always do some warmup exercises.

- Start with a lightweight kettlebell if you are new to this exercise.

- Avoid hinging at your lower back. It may lead to serious injuries to your back. Always hinge at the hips.

Benefits of Kettlebell Deadlift

- It activates a lot of muscles in your body including the quadriceps, hamstrings, glutes, forearms, core, etc.

- It improves your posture.

- It sculpts your core and body.

- It enhances body awareness and coordination. The dynamic movements of the kettlebell help improve muscle connection and focus of the mind.

- It is highly safe. Kettlebells put less pressure on your spine compared to traditional equipment like barbells.

- It improves grip strength.

Standing-Back-Extension

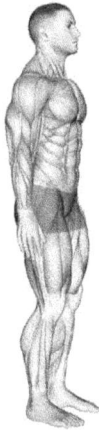

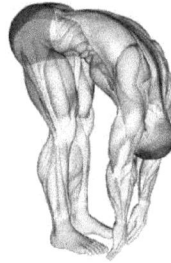

Instructions:

● Stand up tall with your feet together and rotate your hip joint to bend forward.

● While keeping your knees straight, extend your hands to bring your fingertips in line with the tips of your toes.

● Ensure that your knees are not locked. You may bend them slightly to prevent this.

● Keep your quadriceps fully engaged and your legs straight without hyperextending.

● Let your head hang and try to bring your weight into the balls of your feet.

- Pause for a few seconds.

- To return to the starting position, inhale and contract your abdominal muscles as you rise slowly.

- Repeat as many times as you can.

Body form mistakes to avoid

- Rounding your upper back

- Rolling your shoulders forward

- Locking your knees

- Rounding your lower back

Hip raise

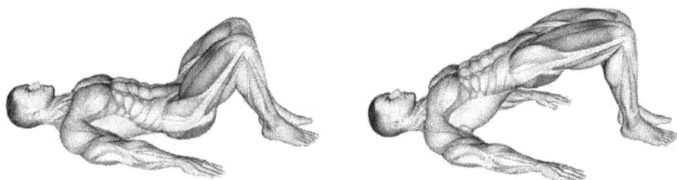

Instructions:

• Start by lying down with your back on the floor with your knees bent, your feet flat on the floor and shins vertical.

• Rest your hands on the floor at your sides with your palms flat for stability.

• Lift your hips off the floor by pushing your feet into the floor while engaging your glutes and back muscles.

• Keep extending your hips upward while pushing down through your heels until they align with your shoulders and knees. Hold that position for 2 seconds.

• Slowly lower your hips back to the floor in a controlled motion to return to the starting position.

3. The Push-up

The push-up is one of the most basic bodyweight exercises that can help you build your upper body strength, muscle mass, and pressing performance. It targets muscles in the chest, arms, and shoulders. It also reinforces the core and helps build stabilizer muscles throughout your body.

Advantages of Push-ups

• You do not require any equipment to do push-ups. You can do them anywhere, anytime.

• They are easy to learn.

• They are simple to perform.

• They are foundational upper body hypertrophy exercises to develop the chest, triceps, and anterior shoulder.

• You can use them to establish control and strength necessary for more advanced exercises.

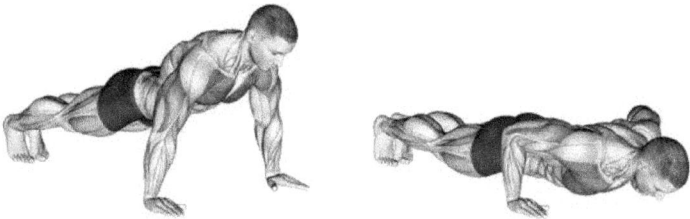

Instructions:

• Start in a high plank position with the back straight. Your hands should be a bit wider than shoulder-width apart, palms flat, fingers spread and pointing forward. Keep your abs tight, butt squeezed, and back flat. Engage your core and glutes. Your legs should be fully extended behind with feet and thighs actively pressed together. Keep your head neutral so that your entire body is straight.

• Pull your shoulder blades together to create tension in your upper back. This ensures proper stability while lowering yourself down.

• Next, bend your elbows and lower your body until your chest touches the floor. Your head and shoulders should not slouch forward towards the floor. Ensure that your thighs, hips, and chest make contact on the floor at the same time. Your entire body should maintain a straight line. To help maintain a neutral neck, gaze at a spot that is a foot or two in front of you. Keep your elbows tucked in close and parallel to your body.

• Once you touch the floor, push through your palms and press yourself away and upwards to return to the starting position.

Body form tips when performing push-ups

• Never round your back. Keep your back straight throughout the move.

• Engage your muscles even in the lowering phase.

• Always keep your abs and butt tight to brace your core during the push-ups.

- Push your weight through your entire hand, including the fingers. This helps prevent straining your wrist.

- Remember to breathe during the movements.

- Stop immediately you realize that your form is being compromised.

Alternative push exercises

You can try easier variations like knee push-ups, wall push-ups, and incline push-ups if you are a beginner or have physical limitations that might impair this move. And if you get stronger as you progress and feel like you need something harder to challenge your muscle strength, try to decline push-ups.

Knee push-up

Knee push-ups are done the same way as push-ups but on your knees.

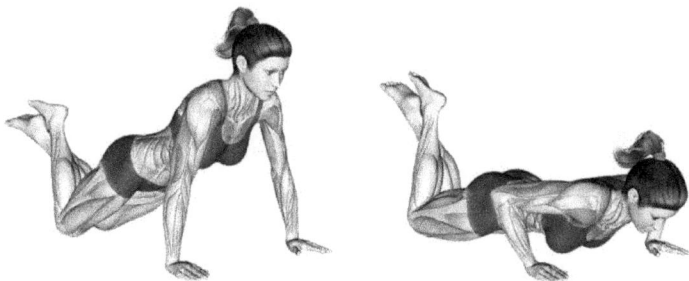

Instructions:

- Start by kneeling on the floor.

- Extend your arms on the floor in front of you. Your hands should be shoulder-width apart, palms flat, fingers spread and pointing forward.

- Keep your abs tight as you bend your elbows and lower your torso until your chest touches the floor.

- Push through the palms of your hand and press your torso away and upwards to return to the starting position. The movement should be slow and steady. Don't rush your body.

- Perform 10-15 reps.

Incline push-up

For this, you need a sturdy box, bench, or table.

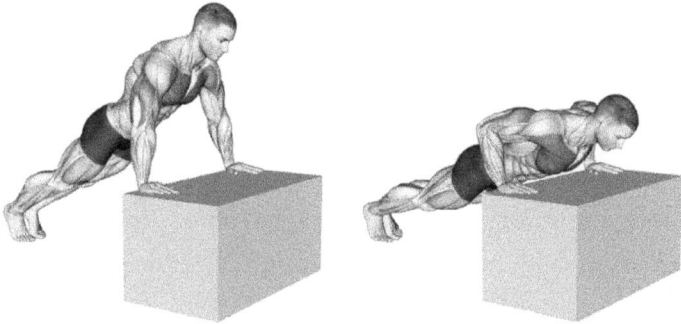

Instructions:

● Stand facing the box, bench, or table then bend down and place both hands on the edges of the box. Make sure that your hands are a tad wider than shoulder-width apart.

● Keep your arms straight (don't lock your elbows) and align your feet to ensure that your body is completely straight. (Your head should be in-line with your spine)

● Next, bend your elbows and slowly lower your chest towards the edge of the box as you breathe in. Keep your body straight and rigid.

- Exhale as you push yourself up by straightening your arms until your elbows are fully extended, but not locked.

Form mistakes to avoid

- **Placing your hands too wide**. This reduces the range of motion of the exercises, reducing the overall effectiveness of the move.

- **Poor alignment.** Your entire body should be straight. Don't slump, sag, or bend your hips or knees. Your upper and lower body should be in straight alignment.

- **Shorter range of motion.** Take this movement through your full range of motion at each rep, right from straight arms to fully bent arms. If you are a beginner and you achieve the full range, opt for wall push-ups.

Wall Push-ups

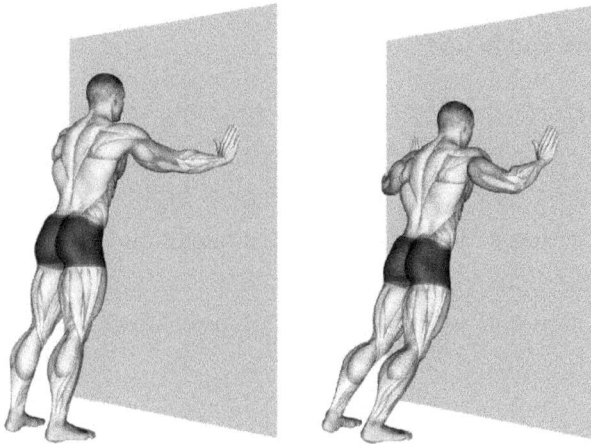

Instructions:

● Facing a wall, stand just a few feet from it.

● Lean in slightly and place your hands on the wall at chest level, a tad wider than shoulder-width apart.

● Inhale as you bend your elbows and lower body towards the wall, slowly and deliberately. Pull your abs in and maintain a straight back.

● Move until your elbows are at 90-degree angle.

● Exhale as you slowly and deliberately push off the wall back to the starting position.

- Repeat as many times as you can to build strength and endurance.

Decline Push-ups

To perform this exercise, you're going to need a raised surface like a bench or box as you did with incline push-ups. Remember, when the surface is higher, the exercise will be hard. So, if you are completely new to this exercise then you will need to start with a low surface like a step and work your way up over time.

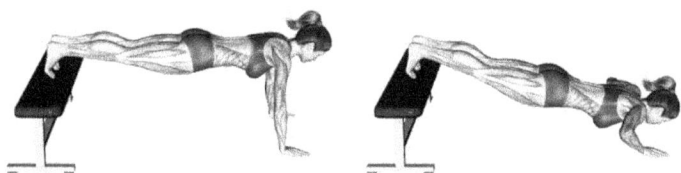

Instructions:

- Start by getting down on all fours in front of the elevated surface. Put your hands on the floor a bit wider than shoulder-width apart with fingers facing forward.

- Carefully extend your legs one at a time to put your feet on the elevated surface.

- Brace your core and straighten your elbows so that your entire body straightens up and forms a long line from the top of your head to your heels. This is where your movement starts or what we call the starting position.

- Next, take a deep breath and bend your elbows to push yourself back into the floor in a slow and controlled motion until your arms form 90-degree angles.

- From this point, breathe out and extend your arms by pushing through your palm to return to starting position.

Pike Push-up

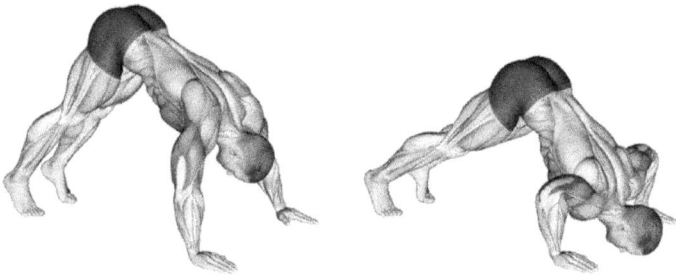

Instructions:

- Start in a downward dog position on the floor. Your hands should be shoulder-width apart and planted firmly on the floor. Your arms and legs should be straight with toes firmly pressed into the floor. Your body should form an upside-down V.

- Make sure that your head is in line with your arms and heels slightly raised off the ground. Then, bend your elbows slowly as you lower your upper body until your forehead nearly touches the ground. Ensure that your legs remain straight.

- Pause for 1 or 2 seconds and then straighten your arms and push yourself back up to the starting position.

- This completes one rep.

Form tips

- Your head should not touch or hit the floor but try to get it as close to the floor as possible.

- Push slowly to avoid slipping or falling on your face or injuring your shoulders.

Elevated pike push-ups

This move is similar to pike push-ups, the only difference is elevating your legs to make it a bit harder.

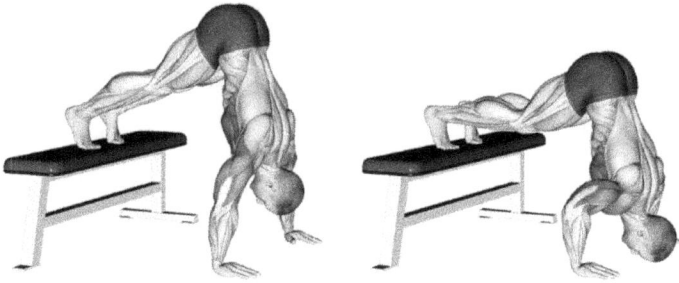

Instructions:

● Get into the pike position with your feet elevated on a bench. Your hands should be shoulder-width apart and planted firmly on the floor. Your arms and legs should be straight with toes firmly pressed onto the bench.

● Bend your elbows slowly as you lower your upper body until your forehead nearly touches the ground.

● Pause for 1 second then push through your hands and return to the starting pike position.

4. The Vertical Press

Vertical pressing is simply pushing a weight in a straight line up and overhead. All the exercises that use this movement pattern can be performed using free weights like dumbbells and kettlebells or body weight. My recommendation is the kettlebell single-arm military press.

Kettlebell one-arm military press

This can be done standing or sitting, but for this purpose, I am showing you the standing version.

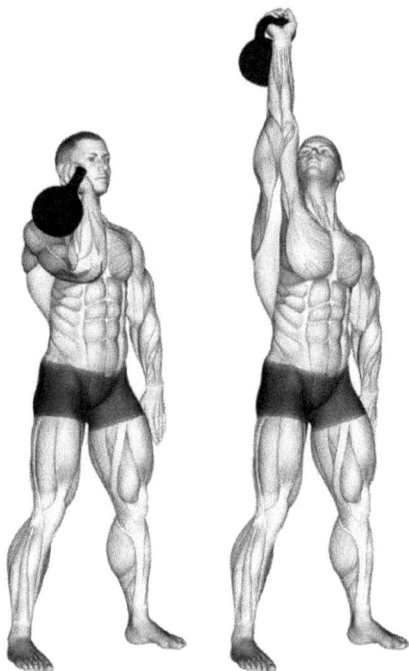

Instructions:

• Start by standing upright with a kettlebell right in front of you. Extend your legs and hips to grab the kettlebell with your right hand and bring it to your shoulder such that the kettlebell is just above your shoulder. As you raise the kettlebell, rotate your wrist so your palm faces inwards. Keep your wrist strong and straight, don't bend it. The kettlebell should also rest comfortably in the crook of your elbow around chest high. This is the starting position.

• Squeeze your butt and brace your core to help stabilize your body.

• Without bouncing or bending your knees, raise the kettlebell straight up overhead. Ensure that your wrist remains locked in a straight line. Stay in this position for 1 or 2 seconds.

• Slowly and gently lower the kettlebell in a controlled motion back to the starting position.

• Repeat the movements for a full set and then switch to the left hand.

Alternative vertical press exercises

Try these out from time to time because different techniques recruit different parts of the same muscles, and it is also fun to modify your workouts.

Standing kettlebell Arnold press

Named after Arnold Schwarzenegger, this is a slight variation on the military press but always done in a standing position. This exercise works the anterior delts more.

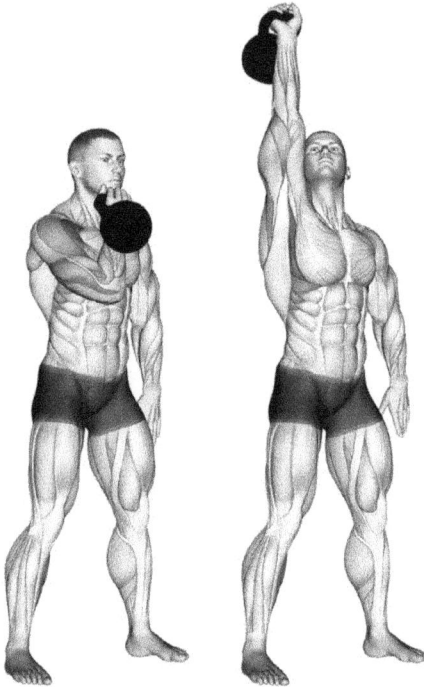

Instructions:

• Select a kettlebell that you can comfortably lift without straining but still feel the workout. Not too light nor too heavy. Choose the one that can allow you to comfortably perform around 10 reps.

- Place the kettlebell on the floor, right in front of you.

- Extend your legs and hips to grab the kettlebell. Use one hand to lift the kettlebell to your front delts such that it rests directly below your chin. Your arm should be at the top of a biceps curl position with your palm facing inwards. This is the starting position.

- Keep your wrist strong and straight, your elbow tucked into your sides.

- Brace your core and keep your shoulders down and tight.

- Open the arm and raise the kettlebell straight up overhead and retract your shoulders.

- Press the kettlebell overhead. As you lift the kettlebell overhead, rotate your wrist so that your palm is facing away from you and pause for a second or two to put tension on your delts.

- Slowly lower the kettlebell in a controlled motion back to the starting position and rotate your wrist so that your palm faces you.

If you are a beginner or have physical limitations that might impair this movement, try easier variations like a light shoulder press. You can also try bodyweight alternatives like pike push-up and bench pike push-up if you want to make it harder.

Light shoulder press (1-5 lb. weight)

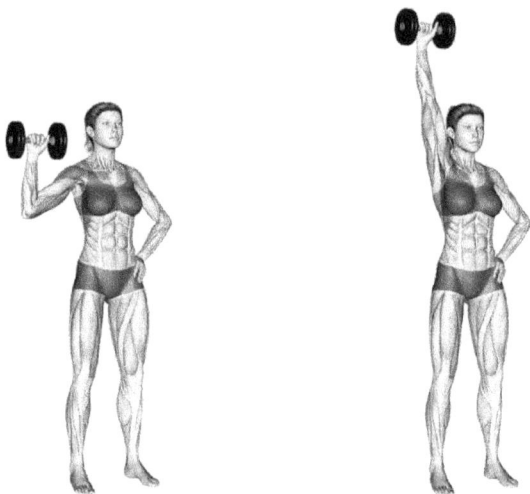

Instructions:

• Grab a dumbbell in one hand and stand tall with your legs shoulder-width apart.

• The arm holding the dumbbell should be bent at about a 60-degree angle such that the dumbbell rests slightly above your shoulder with your palm facing the front.

• Keep your core braced and extend through your elbow to lift the dumbbell directly above your head. Press it over your head until your arm is almost completely locked out.

● Pause for a second or two and then slowly lower the weight back down to your shoulder in a controlled motion.

● Repeat for the recommended number of reps.

5.   The Pull

Pulling exercises can be done both horizontally and vertically, just like pushing exercises. Some of the horizontal pulling exercises include rows. Also, just like the push, the pull exercises contribute to overall upper body strength.

The most famous pulling exercises are pull-ups, but I prefer replacing them with a single-arm kettlebell row because not everyone has a pull-up bar installed at home, and not every beginner can perform several pull-ups in good form. All in all, both exercises are great.

Single-arm Kettlebell Row

The primary muscles worked by this exercise include your back, posterior deltoid, lats, rhomboids, traps, and biceps.

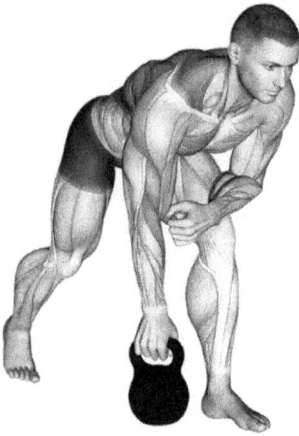

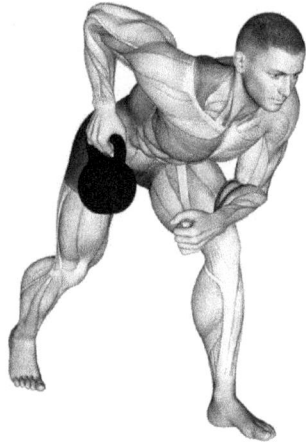

Instructions:

- Stand upright with the kettlebell in front of you.

- With your legs hip-width apart, take a large step forward with your left leg to position your legs in a split stance.

- Slightly bend over to get in a starting position. Your right leg and back should remain straight. Bend your left knee to form a 90-degree angle.

- Rest your left elbow on your left knee for stability. Make sure you maintain a neutral spine.

- Extend your right hand and grab the kettlebell with a neutral grip. This is the starting position.

- Breathe out, bend your elbow, retract your shoulder blade, and pull the kettlebell up towards your stomach. Maintain a straight back.

- Inhale as you extend your right hand to lower the kettlebell back to the starting position and repeat.

- Perform all the repetitions recommended for the right side before switching to the left side.

<u>Alternative pull exercises</u>

Pull-up

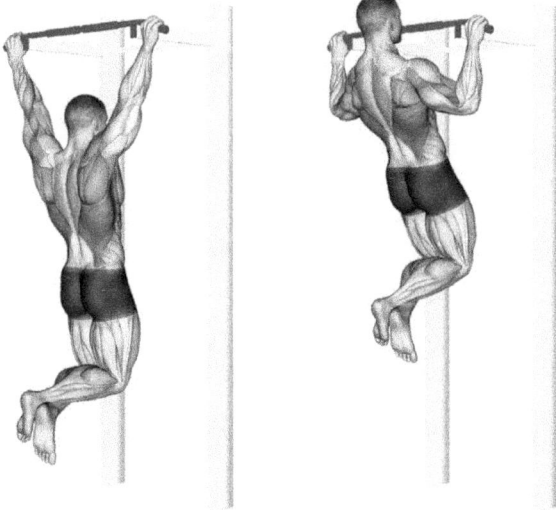

Instructions:

- Start by standing tall, facing a pullup bar.

- Grip the bar about shoulder-width apart and your palms facing away from you.

- Hang from the bar with your arms fully extended. This is the starting position.

- Pull yourself up. Squeeze your lats hard, bend your elbows pulling them down towards the floor to raise yourself up.

- Pull yourself up until your chin passes the bar.

- Pause for a second then slowly lower yourself back to the starting position.

- This completes one rep.

If you are a beginner or have physical limitations, you may try pull variations like negative pull-ups, TRX rows, or doorway rows.

Total Resistance Exercises (TRX)

I have tried TRX belts and resistance bands for my workouts but I did not like them because I could not train all my muscle groups effectively. However, these accessories can be very helpful when training your back and you do not have a pull-up bar installed. With them you can do standing row:

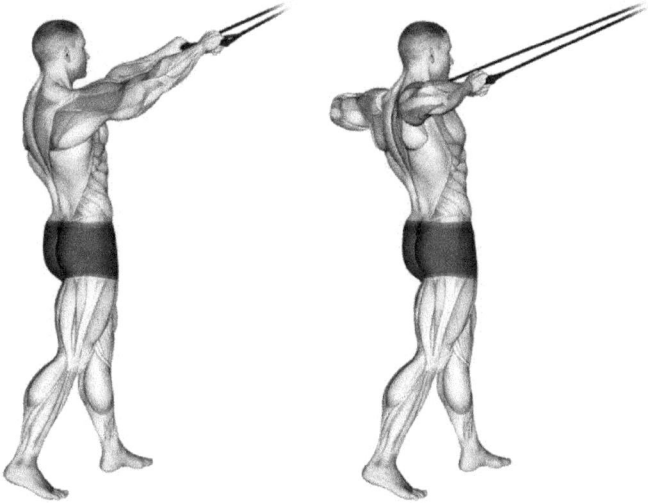

Instructions:

● Hook the TRX cable/resistance bands up on something high so that its handles hang at chest height.

● Stand with your legs hip-width apart and grab the handles with both hands. Your palms should face each other.

- Lean back and extend your arms out to take your weight. The closer your feet are to the anchor the harder the move.

- Pull yourself up to the handles so that the handles end up right under your chest.

- Hold this position for one second then inhale as you slowly lower yourself back in a controlled motion until you're fully extended again.

- This completes the first rep.

Door-way Rows

When you are traveling or do not have any resistance training equipment, you can do this simple bodyweight row in a doorway.

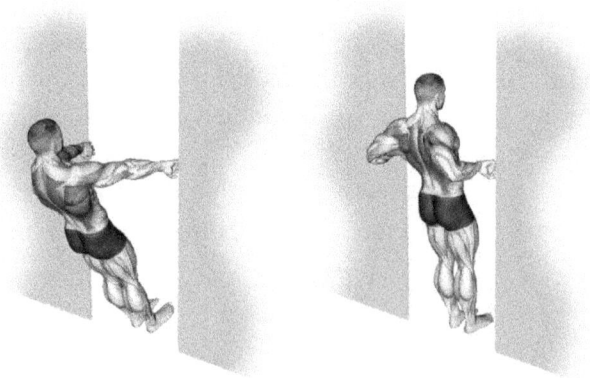

Instructions:

- Open the door that you want to use.

- Stand in the doorway with your feet a few inches inside the frame.

- Grab onto its side frames with both hands at a chest level.

- Bend your legs a little bit and lean back until your arms are fully extended. Your back should be straight.

- Bend your arms and pull yourself towards the door until your chest nearly touches the door frames.

- This completes one repetition.

Inverted Row Under Table

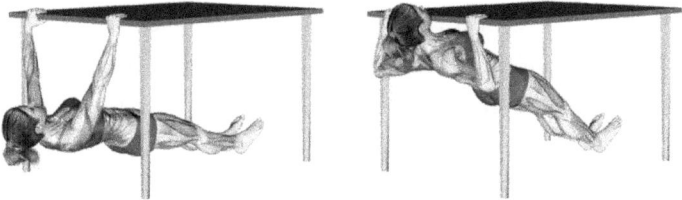

Instructions:

- Start by lying down under a solid table with your hands vertical to its edge.

- Extend your arms fully and grab the edge of the table with an overhand grip. Your hands should be a tad wider than shoulder-width apart. The fingers should be on the surface of the table.

- Your feet should touch the ground at the heels. Make sure that your body is suspended or slightly off the ground. Your heels should be the only part of your body in contact with the floor.

- Brace your core and tighten your glutes to engage your lower back. Ensure that your body is in a straight line from your torso to your feet.

- Pull yourself up, leading with your chest until it touches the table. Keep your body straight, your core braced, and glutes tight throughout the movement. Don't let your hips sink down.

- Hold this position for a second while ensuring your shoulder blades are retracted then slowly lower yourself back to the starting position.

Keep in mind that you will need some experience to carry your weight with your fingertips and to perform row movement using body weight. I prefer doing this exercise using a parallel bar.

6. The Core

Your core is made up of a set of complex muscles that work in tandem to stabilize and flex the spine and run the entire length of the torso on both anterior and posterior sides.

When you correctly perform the major compound exercises, you engage your core muscles a lot. This is why most people think that they don't need to perform core exercises.

The truth of the matter is, compound exercises don't work your core muscles as much as people think, even if you perform them with heavy loads. Research even confirms this. That's why you need to do quite a bit of exercise that targets your core to achieve the look that you really want. I recommend the following moves to strengthen your core.

Leg Raises

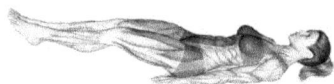 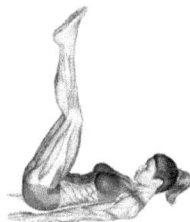

Instructions:

• Lie on your back with your legs straight and feet together. Your arms should be placed by your sides with palms facing down.

• Engage your core and keep your legs straight as you lift them a few inches off the floor. Your toes should be pointed away from your body, your pelvis slightly tucked in and your ribs down. Remember to tuck in your chin throughout the movement. This is the starting position.

• While maintaining that alignment, raise your legs towards the ceiling by flexing your hips until they are completely flexed. Your legs should form a 90-degree angle with your upper body.

• Hold at the top of the movement for one second.

• Then slowly lower your legs back down until they are just above the ground.

• Hold this position for a second, then release.

• Repeat for the recommended number of reps.

Alternative core exercises

Hanging leg raise

Not every beginner can do this exercise correctly and you also need a pull-up bar to perform it, but I believe it is the most effective exercise to train all parts of your abs.

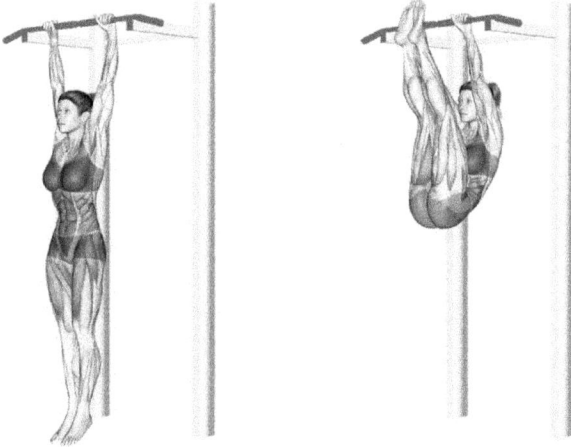

Instructions:

● Start by grabbing a pull-up bar with an overhand grip. Ensure to wrap your thumbs around the bar for improved stability.

● Tighten your abs and hip flexors to engage your core and tilt your pelvis slightly behind.

- Lift your feet off the ground and raise your straight legs toward in front of you. Exhale during this phase of the movement.

- Continue raising your legs as far as you can as long as you can keep a good form. Aim at getting them parallel to the ground or a little higher if possible.

- Hold that position for one second then inhale as you lower your legs back slowly to return to the starting position. This completes one rep.

The Crunch

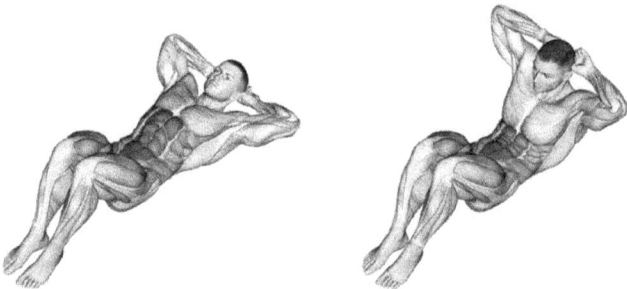

Instructions:

- Lie on your back with knees bent, feet flat on the floor, and hip-width apart.

- Place your hands behind your head with fingers interlocked and bend the elbows out to the sides.

- Brace your core and draw your navel towards your spine. Tilt your chin slightly, ensuring there is some space between it and your chest. This is the starting position.

- Exhale as you curl up and forward so that your head, neck, and shoulder blades lift off the floor.

- While breathing continuously, hold at the top of the movement for a few seconds, and then lower yourself slowly back to the starting position.

- Repeat while ensuring perfect form for each rep.

The Plank

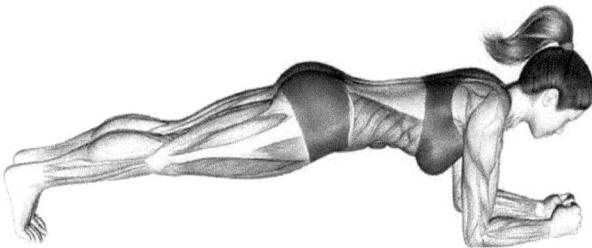

Instructions:

- Start by getting down on all fours with elbows planted directly under your shoulders, toes grounded into the floor, and your forearms facing forward. Keep your head relaxed and neutralize your neck and spine by gazing at a spot on the floor about a foot in front of your hands.

- Engage your core and abdominal muscles and pull your navel inwards. Keep your torso straight and tight. Your entire body should be in a straight line, from your head to your toes.

- Hold this position for at least 15 seconds, then release your body to the floor.

- Increase the holding time as you get more comfortable with the move.

Common form mistakes

To get the most out of your plank exercise and avoid straining your muscles and injuring yourself, avoid the errors below:

- Arching your back. An arched back prevents you from engaging your abdominal muscles thus putting more of your weight onto your arms. To avoid this, keep your shoulders down and wide.

- Sagging your hips. This happens once your abs reach their fatigue limit. And this means you should end the plank. If your hips start sagging at the beginning, try to separate your feet a bit wider and concentrate on tightening your abs.

- Tilting your head up. Avoid tilting your neck. Keep it neutral and in line with the body. Gaze at a spot on the floor to prevent this.

And these are the six most important compound exercises. Just follow all the instructions keenly and be sure of what you're doing. To help you gain the most out of these exercises, see more tips and the factors to consider in the next chapter.

Chapter 5: The Principles of Weight Training

"There's more to life than training, but training is what puts more in your life."
~ Brooks Kubik

Strength training is not just about finding weights and pumping iron. There are several techniques that you need to master before you start strength training. In this chapter, we are going to discuss all the factors that you need to consider before you begin your strength training program. Read on!

Training Frequency

How often you work out can vary depending on, among other factors, your training goals and the level of training. Regular strength training puts stress on your muscles and produces some degree of tissue microtrauma (temporary weakness in muscle cells that stimulates tissue-building processes and strength development).

After every exercise, tissues respond to the training stimulus by rebuilding. This results in stronger and larger muscles. This process of tissue-building typically takes from one day up to a week. Although your training frequency may vary, most experts recommend training most major muscle groups once every 3 to 5 days.

The higher the intensity and volume of individual workouts, the less frequently you can do them to have plenty of recovery time. You also need to take some days off from exercising to give your muscles time to recover fully. I always aim to rest for at least 2 days (48 hours) to ensure full recovery.

If you can lift weights three days per week - training for three nonconsecutive days a week with rests in between (e.g., Monday-Wednesday-Friday) ensures consistency and produces excellent results. But research shows that strength training for two days a week (for example, Mondays and Thursdays) produces nearly the same muscle development effect as three days of strength training workouts per week (Westcott, 2015). Because of that, it is my recommended option to have the best results with the least amount of effort:

Monday	Tuesday & Wednesday	Thursday	Friday, Saturday & Sunday
Workout	2 days off	Workout	3 days off

So, whether you train for two or three days a week, your rate of muscle development should be the same because training frequency isn't as important as challenging your muscles enough during each workout and having enough rest between workouts.

You can also gain strength by training for only one day a week, but research shows that such frequency helps to maintain your muscle but reduces your muscle development rate by about 50% (Westcott et al. 2009).

Some people train muscle groups in splits and go to the gym three to six times per week. That's completely fine. You can even do one total body workout every two weeks if your goal for strength training is to maintain your strength and muscle.

I advise against missing your workout for two weeks, and suggest doing 1-3 workouts a week to remain consistent.

Remember, consistency is as important as frequency. Missing the workout sessions on your schedule is unproductive, and training your muscles without sufficient recovery to make up for missed days is counterproductive.

Therefore, it is important to establish a regular every-other-day, every-other-two days, or every-other-week strength training schedule that is compatible with your goals, recovery, and lifestyle and includes one to three days of training each week.

Sets and Reps

An exercise set refers to a series of repetitions performed sequentially in an exercise. For instance, if you pick up a kettlebell and perform eight military presses, you've completed one set of 8 repetitions. If you take a rest and then repeat this procedure, you would have completed 2 sets of 8 repetitions.

If you are a beginner in a strength training program, you should perform one set of each exercise. Research shows that people starting on strength training can gain the same muscle improvement benefits by performing one set per exercise as they would by performing three sets.

This is because muscles respond faster to resistance exercises in untrained individuals as their level of strength is low. This leaves room for improvement. Additionally, focusing on performing one set of each exercise at the beginning helps you master the moves and avoid injuries.

The good news is that this immediate and significant improvement motivates you to continue working out. However, as time goes by (after three or four months), strength gains levels off. And this is when you need to increase the number of sets and move it to three to five sets per exercise to acquire the desired muscle improvement.

Repetition (reps) refers to the number of times you perform a specific strength training exercise in one set. Ideally, the required number of reps per set is between six and 12. The upper end of this range focuses more on muscle endurance while the lower end focuses more on strength and power.

Your muscles respond differently depending on the kind of stimuli you subject them to, including changing the number of reps performed per set, the weight or load being lifted, the number of sets, time under tension, or the speed at which you perform the exercise.

The most important thing that you need to know about repetitions per set is that you want to reach muscular failure within the 6-12 range depending on your main goal for strength training; whether it is to gain muscle endurance or strength and power.

If your primary goal is to gain power and strength, then you will need to perform between 1-6 reps with a weight that will ensure muscle failure. If you can't do one rep, the weight is too heavy for you. If you can perform more than 6 reps, the weight is too light for power and strength purposes.

If your primary goal for strength training is muscle endurance, then you should be able to perform 12 or more reps. If you can't perform up to the 12th rep, the weight is too heavy for your muscles to endure.

The number of sets performed in an exercise also varies depending on your training goals. According to the National Strength and Conditioning Association (NSCA), below are the suggested range of sets (Kamb, 2021):

• If you want to build muscular endurance, you will need to perform 2-3 sets of 12 to 20+ reps.

• If you want to build muscular hypertrophy, you will need to perform 3-6 sets of 6 to 12 reps.

• If your training goal is to build more muscular strength, then you need to perform 2-6 sets of less than 6 reps.

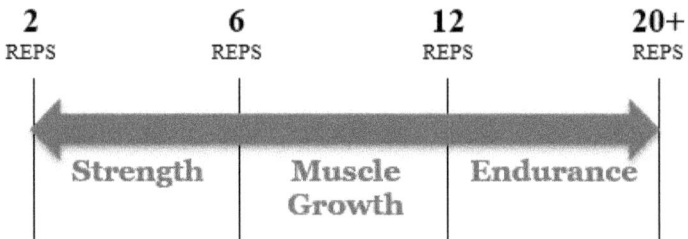

2 REPS	**6** REPS	**12** REPS	**20+** REPS
Strength	Muscle Growth	Endurance	

Keep in mind that these ranges are optimal for building strength or muscle. That does not mean that if you perform 4 sets you will only build strength but not muscle or, if you perform 10 reps that doesn't mean that you will only build muscle, but not strength.

Some studies show that you can gain the same muscles by performing many reps using lighter weights until failure. I prefer using heavier weights and performing fewer reps. For instance, performing 3x10 reps instead of 3x30. This helps save time and to focus better on proper body form and movement techniques.

Based on the above suggestions, I recommend performing 3 sets of 6-12 reps to reap the benefits of both muscle and strength building. Do not forget to pick a weight that is challenging. So, if you can perform more than the maximum number of reps required to achieve a specific goal, it is time that you increase the weight to progress in your workout.

First get a weight that you can lift no more than 6 times. If you are not a beginner, it can take a year or so to do more than 12 reps with this weight and you will need to get a new one. Before increasing the weight, however, you can try other progression methods to advance your workouts.

Repetition Speed

Repetition speed refers to how fast you're lifting and lowering the weight in each repetition (weight, in this case, includes body weight too, and lift also refers to the upward movement of your weight regardless of the direction your body moves). In simple terms, it is the time required to perform each repetition.

The longer it takes to complete a rep or set, the higher the time under tension. If an exercise becomes so easy in a way that you can do more reps than the maximum recommendation, slow down the movement. Take more time to focus as you work your muscles through a full range of motion. This forces your muscles to work harder and optimize muscular strength, endurance, and growth.

To increase time under tension in your workout, decrease your tempo. For instance, if you complete the kettlebell goblet squat with a tempo of 1:1:1, it means that you take one second to lower your body, one second to pause in the squat position, and one second to stand up and return to the starting position.

If you find it so easy to perform, then slow the movement down to a tempo of 2:1:2, 3:1:3…, and so on. When you can complete the exercises using a 5:1:5 tempo comfortably, increase the weight you're using.

To some extent, repetition speed depends on personal preference. Performing repetitions under control is crucial. When we say "under control," we are generally referring to repetition speed without using inertia or momentum (this is not the case for kettlebell swing). Controlled muscular tension challenges your body more and decreases your risk of injury.

One of the best ways to assess your repetition speed is the stop test. Try stopping the repetition at any point in the movement range during a repetition. If you can stop, then you are using the right repetition speed..

Exercise Load/Weight

The selection of an appropriate exercise resistance or load is the first safety concern for anyone participating in strength training. The most important thing is to ensure that your starting weight is not too heavy. The number of repetitions performed in an exercise set is largely determined by the weight you lift or the amount of resistance you use.

If your main goal is muscle strength, you will need to lift a weight that will allow you to complete 1-6 reps comfortably. Continue training with these weights until you can perform more reps with the same load, then increase or manipulate the resistance following the overload principle.

Rest Periods Between Sets and Exercises

A rest period is the time spent resting between sets to allow your muscles some time to recover. The rest period between sets is usually between 30 seconds and 2 minutes (Rogers, 2020). So, when you're performing two or more sets of the same exercise, allow your muscles to recover for 1-2 minutes between sets. This time is sufficient to restore most of the energy used in performing the movements and recover your muscles.

To reduce the overall effects of fatigue on subsequent muscular efforts, you need to take a brief rest between successive exercises. 1-2 minutes of rest between different exercises is usually enough.

In general, the rest time between exercise sets falls between the following ranges for different training goals:

- If you want to build muscle strength, the rest interval between sets is 2 to 5 minutes.

- If you want to increase muscle endurance, the rest interval between your sets during an exercise is 30-60 seconds.

- If your goal for training is muscle hypertrophy, then the rest interval between your exercise sets should be 30 to 90 seconds.

| 30 | 60 | 90 | 2 | 5 |
| SEC | SEC | SEC | MIN | MIN |

Muscle Growth

Muscle Growth

Strength

Endurance

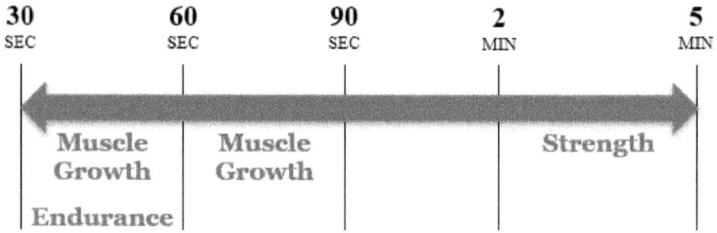

After performing your exercise, rest until you regain your normal breathing before moving to the next. That's what I do. I don't necessarily time myself to ensure that I am resting for exactly 1-2 minutes between my exercises.

Breathing Pattern

Never hold your breath during strength training, regardless of the type and intensity of the exercise you are performing. Holding your breath can cause excessive internal pressure that may restrict blood flow. This may result in symptoms like lightheadedness and high blood pressure responses, interfering with your workout. To prevent these undesirable effects, breathe continuously throughout your exercise sets.

Always exhale during the most difficult phase of the repetition (difficult lifting, pushing, or pulling), sometimes referred to as sticking point, and inhale during the easier lowering or return phase of each repetition. This helps maintain a more desirable internal pressure response. Since continuous breathing is an essential element of safe strength training exercises, you are advised to practice proper breathing on every repetition you perform during the entire workout.

Body Form

Correct body posture while working out is more important than the weights you lift and the sets/reps you perform. Perfecting your form during workouts can help up your game and improve your physique. Here are some of the benefits of maintaining good form as you exercise:

• **It helps prevent injuries.** Practicing proper form during your workouts helps you avoid weight and flexibility-related injuries. Weightlifting (whether it is your own body weight, free weight, or any other) puts more stress on your muscles. And since all your body parts are linked to each other, if one part gets out of balance, the rest breaks down. For example, if you squat in a bad form, you risk injuring your back.

• **It helps reduce wasted energy during exercise.** Poor form during a workout forces you to use more effort and unnecessary energy when performing the exercises. If you exercise in proper body form, you may use less energy to perform the same exercise. Your workout becomes smooth and enjoyable too! No straining.

- **It enhances workout effectiveness and efficiency.**
Practicing proper form during an exercise gives you a
functional workout experience. It enables you to move
your joints and muscles through a full range of motion,
experiencing a complete extension and contraction of
muscles and much better results.

Most people do not perform their exercises in proper
form. But you need to know that proper form is an
essential element to achieving your fitness goals. It helps
reduce muscle strains giving you a pain-free
environment to exercise. It also enables you to correctly
work the targeted muscles.

Range of Motion

Range of motion refers to how far you can move your
joints on each rep. In other terms, it refers to your joints'
capability to go through the complete spectrum of the
movements you make during an exercise. Most experts
recommend exercising through the full range of joint
motion.

Full range of motion means exercising from the position
of full muscular stretch to the position of full muscular
contraction. This means that when the target muscle
group is fully stretched, the opposing muscle group is
fully contracted, and vice versa.

A good example is your biceps and triceps; if you move your elbow joint through a full range of motion, your biceps stretch fully while your triceps contract fully. Of course, you shouldn't exceed normal joint limits or feel pain during the movement. Eliminate any exercise that causes joint pain or discomfort, and ensure you train only in a pain-free range of motion.

Having an enormous range of motion in your exercise has the following benefits:

- **Enhances joint flexibility.** Performing your exercises through a full range of motion increases your joint flexibility. Flexibility is very important when it comes to training your body as it also helps with posture and weightlifting during strength training. Therefore, if you want your workout to be more effective and efficient, you have to perform your movement through a full range of motion.

- **Enables you to do more exercises with less effort.** Exercising in a full range of joint motion allows you to perform more challenging exercises with less energy. Studies show that people who exercise their muscles through a full range of motion increase their muscle strength thus being able to lift heavier weights without straining.

• **Enhances development of full-range muscular strength.** Muscle building largely depends on the weights you lift and how you lift them. Studies show that lifting your weight in the full range of joint motion develops strength in all the muscles (Westcott, 2015). A lower range of motion in an exercise lowers muscle tension, hindering muscle growth. Lifting heavier weights activates your muscle fiber, which increases your muscle cells, promoting growth. Therefore, to build muscle strength and power, you need to exercise in the full range of motion.

Exercise Progression

Workout progression is what most of us strive for. However, some always stick to what is more comfortable, i.e., performing the same reps/sets with the same weight. This conflicts with the progressive overload principle which is the main training principle.

The progressive overload principle states that to keep gaining strength and muscle mass or achieve any other exercise-related progress, you need to increase your muscle's working load progressively to continually challenge your body and muscles with new training stimuli.

Remember, not all exercises progress at the same rate. And again, don't pile on the weight too fast or force progress by sacrificing form. You will cause more damage to your body.

To avoid injuries and attain the desired results, it is better to lift a lighter load in a full range of motion reps than performing half sloppy reps with heavier loads. I don't mean that half reps and heavier loads are bad. No. What I mean is that it is proper and safer to nail down your form with the full range version first.

To progress your weight, use a heavier load while keeping the reps, sets, rest period, and tempo the same. For example, if you are currently lifting 50 pounds on a particular exercise, you can lift 52.5 pounds the next time you perform the same exercise. Studies indicate that it is safe and productive to increase your weight load by as little as 2.5 pounds at each level of training progression. However, that is not so simple when you use a single dumbbell or kettlebell, so I prefer other progression methods.

Other Progression Methods

To ensure advancement in your fitness goals, you can incorporate other progression methods:

• **Increasing your sets.** To progress your sets, add one set while retaining the weight and rest period. For example, if you're lifting 50 lbs. on a particular exercise for 3 sets of 10 reps, you can do 4 sets of 10 reps with the same weight next time.

- **Up your reps.** To progress your reps, add one rep to each set while retaining the weight and rest period. For example, if you're lifting 50 lbs. on an exercise for 3 sets of 5 reps, you can try to do 3 sets of 6 reps with the same weight next time.

- **Decreasing your rest time.** When decreasing your rest between sets, try to maintain the weight and reps/sets. This makes the exercise more challenging. For instance, if you currently rest for 2 minutes between sets when performing a particular exercise, try dropping the rest time to 1 minute and 30 seconds while lifting the same weight for the same number of sets and reps.

During strength training, how we execute our exercises matters most. To reap the physical and mental benefits of your workout, you need to consider all the factors discussed above. You should be mostly concerned with performing the exercises provided correctly to build the muscle memory and pathway required for long-term results. And for you to achieve this, just follow the advice and suggestions presented in this book.

With a practical understanding and appreciation of these training principles, I believe you're now prepared to follow a simple workout program that I have designed for you in the next chapter. Remember, you need the right training intensity to keep improving in your workouts and this intensity is affected by the principles above.

Key Takeaways

- Use proper form/posture when doing your workout. When lifting weights, ensure that you move your joints through a full range of motion.

- Never hold your breath while exercising. It is advisable to exhale during the most difficult phase of the repetition (difficult lifting, pushing, or pulling), and inhale during the easier lowering or return phase of each repetition.

- Rest for 1-2 minutes between sets and exercises to give your muscles time to recover.

- Perform 3 sets of 6-12 reps of each exercise to reap the most benefits from your workouts.

- Aim for 2 workouts a week and you will have the best results with the least amount of effort.

Chapter 6: The Ultimate Workout Plan

"What makes a weightlifting program successful? Your hard work and dedication."

~Greg Everett

Exercises don't become a workout unless they are planned and arranged into a program, and a workout program cannot help you achieve your training goals smoothly unless the program itself is easy to follow, innovative, and effective.

And in this chapter, I have done just that. But before we get started on the training program, let's explore workout warmup and cool down. We are also going to perform our exercises in super sets, and I am sure you would love to know what they are and why we're using them in our program.

Warm Up and Cool Down

Sometimes, it can be tempting to skip warming up, especially when you are chasing time or just anxious to start your workout. However, warming up before engaging in strenuous physical activity has physiological and psychological benefits.

Strength training places relatively heavy demands on your musculoskeletal system. Therefore, it is very important to warm up before jumping into a strength workout. Activities like jogging in place, brisk walking, and jumping rope are great ways for quickly warming up for your workout. It should take you only 2-5 minutes to perform these warm-up exercises.

Benefits of warming up

- **Lowers the risk of injury.** The last thing that should happen to you after working out is sustaining sprains, strains, or other forms of injuries. Warming up your muscles helps improve their elasticity, reducing the chances of hurting yourself or overheating during exercise.

- **Prepares you mentally for what is ahead.** When your workout gets difficult, it can be very easy to get demotivated and give up. However, if you warm up before the workout, you are less likely to do so. This is because as you warm up, your brain focuses on your body and the physical activity, which carries over into your training session.

- **Increases flexibility.** Warm ups relax your muscles, making it easier to move and execute your workout properly.

- **Improves your blood flow and oxygen.** A five-minute warm-up with an easygoing activity like jogging in place opens blood vessels, improving blood flow to your skeletal muscles. This helps supply your muscles with the required amount of oxygen during exercise, preventing what we sometimes call "oxygen debt."

Cooling down after your workout is as important as warming up. The main aim of cooling down is to gradually bring your heart rate and blood pressure back to normal after the workout. This period is essentially a warm-up in reverse.

During workout, your heartrate is higher than normal, and it is very important to ease it back to normal slowly rather than stopping abruptly.

The cool-down is particularly important for older adults because it prevents the accumulation of blood and other body fluids in the lower legs which could cause undesirable changes in blood pressure, increasing the risk of cardiovascular complications.

A five- to ten-minute cool-down activity like brisk walking followed by stretching exercises facilitates a smooth return to normal blood circulation and heart rate.

Importance of cooling down

• **It aids muscle recovery.** After an intense exercise, lactic acid builds up in your musculoskeletal system. It takes time for this lactic acid to be cleared out of your body. So, cool down exercises facilitate the release and removal of lactic acid, enhancing speedy muscle recovery.

- **Lowers DOMS (Delayed Onset Muscle Soreness).** Although it is normal to experience muscle soreness after a workout, DOMS can create discomfort and prevent you from exercising in the future. Research shows that cooling down after a workout helps alleviate excessive muscle soreness, making you feel more comfortable and ready for the next workout.

Stretching

Even if you don't exercise often, it is important to incorporate stretching into your daily routine. It keeps your muscles flexible and able to perform their full range of motion. The American College of Sports Medicine recommends stretching each of your major muscle groups at least twice a week for 60 seconds per stretch (Collins, 2012).

Should you stretch before working out?

You should not perform static stretching before you exercise. There is no proof that static stretching before exercise can help prevent injury, curb muscle soreness after exercise, or improve your performance. In fact, research shows that performing static stretching alone before working out can decrease your muscle strength and power and weaken your performance (Simic, 2013).

Instead, you should warm up by doing dynamic stretches.

Should you stretch after working out?

This is the best time to stretch. Performing static stretching after exercise helps you cool down, recover, and get ready for the next exercise. Stretching at this time will help improve blood flow, helping deliver nutrients and oxygen to the affected muscles, and facilitating recovery and rejuvenation. It also helps calm down your nervous system and slow your heart rate.

How to stretch safely

If you have to stretch before your workout, ensure that you are not doing it on completely cold muscles. You need to perform some warm-up activities to help generate heat in your muscles before stretching them. You can do this by shaking parts of your body like your arms, hands, and legs.

If the stretch is static, which is done mostly after a workout, hold it for at least 30 seconds. Give your body time to take in the extension. This is much safer for your tissues. You shouldn't feel pain during any phase of your stretch. If you do, then you are not doing it correctly and you should stop. Take the time to do it correctly.

Supersets

This is simply performing two different exercises back-to-back with minimal rest in between.

The benefits of supersets

• **They save time.** Supersets are great when you're short on time. Completing two different exercises without or with minimal rest intervals makes your workout shorter but more efficient. Using supersets, I can complete a whole-body workout in 30 minutes.

• **Increased intensity.** Supersets enable you to perform more work in less time, which in turn helps you gain more from your workout program.

• **Improves muscle endurance.** Supersets help train your muscles to endure longer periods of stress. This helps you get stronger and to sustain your exercises for longer.

• **They help burn more calories.** Several studies have proven that supersets burn more calories during and after your workout.

• **Enhance active rest.** By using supersets, you work one muscle while the opposing one rests. This maximizes muscle growth while burning body fat.

119

The Program

When it comes to muscle building, one of the most important things you need to be doing is compound exercises - core muscle building movements that were presented in Chapter 4. You need to get stronger at those too.

Doing those exercises consistently in a proven program is essential for your progress, especially if you're over 40 or 50.

It's important to also understand the appropriate frequency of training. Frequency essentially means how often you train a muscle group, and there are various ways to train for building muscle. Each one of them has its own merits.

Bodybuilding magazines often recommend splitting your workout routine, e.g., chest on Monday, back on Tuesday, shoulders on Wednesday, legs on Thursday, and arms on Friday. These are specialized split routines that mean you train your chest on Monday and then you don't hit chest again for five to seven days. That is not the most optimal way for most of us to train. I suggest adopting a higher frequency of training with lower sets per session. This means that instead of doing a lot of sets on Monday, divide the sets to two to three workouts by training chest two to three times per week with sufficient rest between your workouts.

Each time you train a muscle, days after the training session you get this protein synthesis muscle building stimulus and that only lasts for a couple days and then you need to train again to get that stimulus. If we slammed our chest with 20 sets, we're not getting more protein synthesis than if we just did several hard sets. Performing 20 sets per muscle group just creates the need for time for recovery. Then we can't train again for another five to seven days.

As we get into our 40s and 50s, it's essential to spread out that volume using two to three full body workouts, using compound exercises spaced throughout the week. This is done to achieve the optimal number of sets and have enough time to recover. When you're hitting the body more frequently, the muscle building stimulus remains constant.

In the program below, I have combined exercises that are highly effective on their own. This program maximizes this effectiveness while minimizing the effort required, leaving you with amazing results. And the best part is, you can do this workout with one weight (either one kettlebell or one dumbbell).

FULL BODY WORKOUT
(WITH SUPERSETS)

1st SUPERSET	
Push-Up	3 sets of 10-20 reps
Kettlebell Goblet Squat	3 sets of 6-10 reps
2nd SUPERSET	
Right arm Kettlebell row	3 sets of 6-10 reps
Left arm Kettlebell row	3 sets of 6-10 reps
3rd SUPERSET	
Right arm Military Press	3 sets of 6-10 reps
Left arm Military Press	3 sets of 6-10 reps
4th SUPERSET	
Kettlebell Swing	3 sets of 6-10 reps
Leg Raise or Crunch	3 sets of 10-20 reps

Helpful Tips

Do push-ups and without rest the goblet squats (superset #1). After you complete these 2 exercises 1 time – rest for 1-2 minutes and repeat superset #1. After you do superset #1 3 times– rest for 1-2 minutes and go to supersets #2, #3, and #4. I suggest that you perform 6-12 reps of each exercise.

I have started with push-ups and squats because they are simple, work different muscle groups and give you a very good warm-up. I left swing for the end because this one is the riskiest for beginners and it's best done when you're properly warmed up after the three previous supersets. Although supersets will help you finish your workout faster, you can also do traditional sets: do one exercise for 3 sets with 1-2 minutes rest after every set before moving to the next exercise. These and other fundamental exercises were described in chapter 4. There you will find alternative exercises if you need to replace any of my recommended exercises.

However, it is important to note that there are several ways to structure your training program; my suggestions are not constant. You may modify and adjust it based on your training goals. But, if you want to get great results with the least amount of effort, this can be a great and sustainable workout system for you.

If you don't like performing supersets and prefer to rest before moving to the next set, you can rest for one minute or until you regain your normal breathing after each set. Then move to the next exercise after you have completed three sets of the same exercise.

123

WORKOUT WITHOUT SUPERSETS	
Push-Up	3 sets of 10-20 reps
Kettlebell Goblet Squat	3 sets of 6-10 reps
Right arm Kettlebell row	3 sets of 6-10 reps
Left arm Kettlebell row	3 sets of 6-10 reps
Right arm Military Press	3 sets of 6-10 reps
Left arm Military Press	3 sets of 6-10 reps
Kettlebell Swing	3 sets of 6-10 reps
Leg Raise or Crunch	3 sets of 10-20 reps

If you have a barbell, pull-up bar, or parallels, try to incorporate exercises that use this equipment in your workout. I love taking advantage of this equipment whenever to perform exercises like incline bench press instead of push-ups or pull-ups instead of rows. But don't scratch your head if you can't access this equipment. **The most important thing is to perform the mentioned compound exercises with whatever equipment is at hand or even without one.**

The dumbbell and kettlebell are both solid options for pursuing personal fitness. If you have a pair of dumbbells, you can use them to perform similar compound movements too.

WORKOUT WITH DUMBBELLS	
Dumbbell Chest Press	3 sets of 6-10 reps
Dumbbell Squat	3 sets of 6-10 reps
Dumbbell Shoulder Press	3 sets of 6-10 reps
Bent-Over Dumbbell Row	3 sets of 6-10 reps
Dumbbell Deadlift	3 sets of 6-10 reps
Leg Raise or Crunch	3 sets of 10-20 reps

If you've got some experience with resistance training, or if you're coming back to resistance training after some time away, intermediate workout routine with free weights will probably be the best fit for you.

Can beginners train with kettlebells and dumbbells?

Yes, absolutely. Beginners can train with free weights, but it's worth noting that form should take precedence when using them for the first few workouts. If you're very new to exercise, recovering from an injury, prefer low-intensity strength training, or have physical limitations that might impair movement, I recommend

125

starting with beginner workout routines using lighter weights, resistance bands, or only bodyweight exercises.

Bodyweight or resistance bands workouts are great for everyone looking to easily tone their muscle, maintain their strength, and health from the comfort of home or while traveling.

These workouts are an invaluable resource, not only for seniors looking for looking how to improve their strength and body composition, but even for bodybuilders looking for a challenging training session when the gym is inaccessible.

BODYWEIGHT WORKOUT	
Push-Up	3 sets of 10-20 reps
Bodyweight Squat	3 sets of 10-20 reps
Bodyweight Row	3 sets of 6-10 reps
Pike Push-up	3 sets of 6-10 reps
Hip Raise	3 sets of 6-10 reps
Leg Raise or Crunch	3 sets of 10-20 reps

RESISTANCE BAND WORKOUT	
Push-Up with Resistance	3 sets of 10-20 reps
Squat with Resistance	3 sets of 10-20 reps
Resistance Band Rows	3 sets of 6-10 reps
Vertical Press	3 sets of 6-10 reps
Deadlift	3 sets of 6-10 reps
Leg Raise or Crunch	3 sets of 10-20 reps

When you get stronger and feel like you need something harder to challenge your muscle strength, or if you've got experience with bodyweight training or weightlifting and you're looking for more challenging workouts, then advanced exercises with a barbell may be suitable.

Barbell exercises are not for everyone, but a lot of people believe they are the best strength training programs because heavier weights will help you gain muscle and strength faster. While it is possible to progress on most exercises using bodyweight or any equipment, they may be insufficient to achieve progressive overload on exercises like the squat, deadlift, bench press, and dumbbell row after several years of training. If you're an experienced lifter and you want or can go to the gym, these are the best barbell exercises to gain strength and muscle mass.

BARBELL WORKOUT	
Barbell Bench Press	3 sets of 6-10 reps
Barbell Squat	3 sets of 6-10 reps
Barbell Bent Over Row	3 sets of 6-10 reps
Seated Barbell Shoulder Press	3 sets of 6-10 reps
Deadlift	3 sets of 6-10 reps
Hanging Leg Raise or Incline Crunch	3 sets of 10-20 reps

If you're unsure how to perform some exercises – don't worry. To make things simple, I've linked all the workouts in this book to videos that show proper form of each exercise in a downloadable PDF.

To get instant access to it, go to **"Free Bonus Material"** at the end of this book.

Total body workouts are great for building muscle and gaining strength, especially for those on the fringes (the people just beginning their weightlifting journey and those who've already achieved most of their genetic potential for muscle gain).

However, if you found these workouts grueling, unsustainable, or your personal preference is to train different muscle groups on different days, I have a solution for you.

To ensure that every reader finds a plan that suits their individual needs, I have added a bonus chapter on workout splits in the updated edition of this book. At the end of this book, you will find a variety of workout plans catering to different fitness levels, equipment, goals, and preferences.

Key Takeaways

- Always warm-up before starting your workout.

- Using supersets is a great way to save on time.

- Focus on compound movements, not on exercises or equipment.

- From time to time, changing one or another exercise or equipment will make your workouts even more effective and fun.

Chapter 7: Recovery

"If you aren't begging for rest, then you aren't training
your best."
~Unknown

Regular exercise is key to a healthy, strong body and
peak physical fitness. However, if you want to get the
most out of your regular workout, that is, getting into
your desired body shape while avoiding injuries, you
need to allow your muscles adequate time to recover.

Some people spend quality time in gyms or exercise from
home with fancy gym equipment and free weights, but
they still don't see the fruits of their efforts, even if they
go the extra mile by increasing the number of reps/sets
and using proper lifting techniques.

I am sure you may have encountered such people, and
they may have discouraged you in one way or another.
Don't let them discourage you from working out. The
problem is not the workouts. The most possible culprit
here is failure to allow your muscles enough time to
recover.

Most people have the wrong impression of how strength
training helps the body build muscle mass and strength.
They think that muscles build during exercise. That's

why many people tend to overlook the concept of recovery period. You need to understand that muscles don't form during the actual workout period, muscle building occurs during recovery time. That's after the workout.

Neglecting recovery protocol can have negative long-term effects on your muscle health. In this chapter, I am going to discuss the recovery concept, its benefits after exercise, and the ways to recover. Read on!

What is Muscle Recovery?

During strength training, your body uses up the energy stored in your muscles, and as a result, your muscles get fatigued and their strength drops below its baseline. It is during the recovery period that more energy is manufactured and stored in your muscles. Muscle recovery is much more than just allowing your muscles adequate time to stop being sore. Later in this chapter, I am going to show you ways to recover faster.

Importance of muscle recovery

If you think taking a break from working out for a day will set you back, think again. The thing is, after working out, you must give your body sufficient break before you exercise again to allow it to recover from the previous workout.

Most people who train frequently tend to overlook the notion that exercise is stress. But wait…, did this statement confuse you? Don't get confused. This is not the same type of stress that you are thinking of. This is good stress. Exercise stresses your muscles, providing long-lasting benefits.

Any intense exercise creates fatigue, micro-traumas, and tears in your muscles. Muscle soreness and pain are the most common symptoms of this effect. If you don't allow your muscles to heal and recover from this damage, it can prevent your muscles' ability to replenish their glycogen stores.

After exercise, lactic acid accumulates within your body cells. There is scientific evidence that built up lactic acid impairs the electrical stimulus required for muscle contraction. It also impairs your body's ability to generate ATP, which is an essential molecule that plays a big role in repeated muscle contraction.

None of the above sounds beneficial, right? It is until you factor in the recovery period that's when you will enjoy the fruits of your workout efforts. For these micro-traumas and tears to heal, we need to create a healing environment for them. It is through recovery that your body will get rid of lactic acid from your muscles and restore its capacity to produce ATP.

What happens if you don't recover?

For beginners, you won't see positive results from your workout. Overworking your muscles without giving them enough recovery time doesn't yield the desired fitness outcome.

Lack of enough sleep at night is another sign of inadequate recovery after exercise. Overtraining makes it hard for your body to differentiate exercise fatigue from other stressors. As a result, your body enters a chronic dominant state of fight-or-flight, leaving you too wired to sleep.

Another indication of inadequate recovery time from exercise is craving sweet or salty foods. During exercise, most of us sweat a lot and lose electrolytes. This creates electrolyte imbalance in your body, making you crave such foods. Research has also associated lack of muscle recovery with hormonal upset and impaired immune function.

Ways in Which Our Muscles Recover

Stretching, rest, nutrition, hydration, sleep, and massage are the six elements of muscle recovery. Let's take a closer look at each element.

1. Stretching

Stretching is an important aspect of exercise, that's why it is recommended that you include it in your workout routine. Dynamic stretching before a workout keeps your body open, giving your muscles space and flexibility to complete the moves safely and through a full range of motion. This helps reduce the risks of injury, muscle soreness, and tears. On the other hand, stretching after a workout helps heal your muscles and reduce DOMS. (For more information on the benefits of stretching, refer to chapter 6.)

2. Rest Days

If you are following a workout program, people will remind you about your workout days and how you need to exercise regularly. But you will never hear anyone talk about rest. Rest days are as important as workout days.

To achieve your training goals, you must include rest days in your workout routine and adhere to them. They help your body repair and recover faster. As discussed earlier, the process of muscle building takes 2-4 days. And while most experts recommend full-body strength training for 2-3 nonconsecutive days per week, this may vary from person to person. The good news is that there is a way your body communicates when it needs rest.

Signs that you need rest

If you notice any of the following signs, your body needs rest and you should plan a rest day:

- Decreased performance. If you stop seeing progress, or you start having difficulties in carrying out your exercises, take a rest day.

- Lack of sleep. If you can't sleep for at least 7-8 hours every night, take some rest from your workout.

- Sore muscles. Although it is quite common and normal to feel sore after your workout, it shouldn't go for a prolonged period. If the soreness is persistent, it is a sign that your muscles are yet to recover from the previous workouts.

- Pain. Consistent pain in your muscles and joints might be a sign of injury from overuse.

- Muscle fatigue. You need to rest if you feel extremely exhausted.

3. Nutrition

Both exercise and diet contribute in equal proportion to the fitness equation. After a workout, protein intake is key as it helps with refueling and recovery of your muscles. At this point, you already know that muscle contraction from consistent training causes microtrauma and tears to your body muscles. To repair and rebuild these muscles, you will need amino acids. This means you will need to consume protein to help supply your muscles with the amino acid.

Your body uses glycogen to fuel your workouts and by the time you're done, your glycogen stores will have depleted. To replenish your glycogen stores, you need to consume carbs. I will be talking more about nutrition and exercise in the next chapter, so keep reading.

4. Hydration

During exercise, your body loses water and electrolytes through sweating. This may cause dehydration, which may lower your performance. Therefore, you are advised to drink plenty of water before, during, and after the workout to keep your body properly hydrated.

The usual recommendation is drinking at least eight glasses, or two liters, of water. Electrolyte water can be a good option because besides keeping your body hydrated, it also supplies your body with important electrolytes like sodium, calcium, potassium, and magnesium, which also play a role in muscle recovery.

5. Sleep

There are two major stages of sleep: Rapid Eye Movement (REM) and Non-Rapid Eye Movement (Non-

REM). To understand the effect of sleep on muscle recovery, you have to understand what happens in these two phases of sleep.

Rapid Eye Movement (REM) Sleep

This phase of sleep accounts for about 25% of your total sleep. It occurs in cycles of about 1.5–2 hours throughout the night. REM sleep dominates the latter half of your sleeping time. It provides your brain with energy that supports it during waking hours. It also restores your mind.

Non-REM Sleep

This is the most important phase in muscle recovery. It is where deep sleep happens. That's why it is sometimes known as the slow-wave or deep sleep phase. It accounts for about 40% of your total sleep. During this phase, your blood pressure goes down and your breathing becomes slower and deeper.

At this time, there are very few activities going on in your brain because it is resting. As a result, the blood supply to your muscles increases, delivering extra amounts of oxygen and nutrients to your muscles. This enhances faster recovery and muscle growth.

Another important thing that occurs during this phase of sleep is the secretion of growth hormones. As your body enters this phase, your pituitary glands release a shot of growth hormones that stimulate tissue growth and muscle repair. Failing to get enough sleep during the night can result in a sharp decline in the secretion of growth hormones.

Research indicates that deficiency of growth hormones is associated with muscle mass loss and reduced exercise capacity.

Sleep enhances muscle recovery through two different ways: protein synthesis and growth hormone secretion. So, if you want to increase muscle mass and recover faster from your previous workouts, it is important to get at least 7-8 hours of sleep every night.

6. Massage

Massage your muscles after training. Massaging the worked muscles helps relieve the lactic acid built up in the areas. This enhances faster recovery.

7. Sauna

In addition to being a relaxing way to end a workout, saunas do have some health benefits. High-temperature exposure helps blood vessels expand, which improves circulation and lowers blood pressure.

Some athletes use saunas to help with performance and endurance. If you're looking to build strength and power, saunas can help with that too. The length of time you stay in a sauna depends on your comfort level, but most guidelines say 15 minutes is a reasonable time limit for most healthy adults.

Key Takeaways

• The muscles strained during an exercise require enough time to heal and repair, therefore, it is very important to take sufficient rest after your workout. Don't overuse your muscles. Take some quality time to rest. Ensure that you get at least 7-8 hours of sleep at night.

• Drink plenty of water (preferably electrolytes) to keep your body hydrated and replace the electrolytes lost through sweating during exercise. The normal recommendation is at least 8 glasses every day.

Chapter 8: Essential Nutrients

"If we could give every individual the right amount of
nourishment and exercise, not too little and not too
much, we would have found the safest way to health."
~ Hippocrates

Exercise and nutrition go hand in hand. Not only do you
have to exercise if you want to acquire a healthy, strong,
and good looking body, but you must eat right.

Eating right doesn't necessarily mean eating only salads
and tasteless foods. Your diet shouldn't feel more like
self-denial than self-improvement.

What I am trying to say is that you can have a good diet
plan structured from the foods that you love. You don't
need to sacrifice your favorite foods in an obsession with
"clean eating."

The decision on what diet to commit to will depend on
your fitness goal. If your goal is weight loss, you will
have to consume fewer calories, and if your goal is to
gain weight and muscle mass, then you will need more
calorie intake.

It is just simple biology; what I have learned over the
years, however, is that you don't need to starve yourself
for you to lose weight, neither do you have to gorge

yourself every chance you get if you want to gain weight or muscle mass.

You need to know that different people have different body types and different metabolic systems. A diet plan that works for another person may not work for you. Therefore, when setting up an eating routine, structure it off what you are used to.

If you want to lose weight and you eat four meals every day, drop one so that you have three meals a day.

It's about moderate, controlled, planned eating. However, regardless of your training goals, you need to consume as little processed and sugary "foods" as possible.

Some people argue that exercise is the most important while others say that it is not as important as diet and other factors. Some still argue that one is 40 percent and another 60 percent. If you didn't know, diet is 100 percent important.

Exercise is also 100 percent.

Remember there are other factors, but these two are the major ones. Does it sound weird? I know you're confused about the total percentage. Yes, it can go even up to 1000 percent. The point here is this: the building blocks of a great body are more like pillars than puzzle pieces. If you make one too weak, the whole structure collapses. For your body to adapt to your training, you need to support it with proper nutrition. And for you to gain more muscle and strength, you need to train correctly.

If you continue consuming a lot of nutrient-empty calories without the right balance of macronutrients, your strength training efforts will end in frustration.

Micro and Macronutrients

Micronutrients consist of vitamins and minerals. Our bodies require these vitamins and minerals to remain in good health. They help with the regulation of metabolism, heart rate, and bone density.

Macronutrients consist of proteins, carbohydrates, and fats. Our bodies require a balance of both micro and macronutrients to function optimally.

Proteins

Proteins are known for building muscles and gaining strength. As we grow older, our testosterone levels decline, and our muscle mass declines too. As a result, fat can occupy the place of muscle cells, leading to undesirable weight gain or body shape and weak muscles. To increase muscle mass, you need to increase the number of proteins you consume.

As we age, our metabolism becomes slower. Therefore, it is recommended that you consume between 1.2–1.7 grams of protein per kilogram of your body weight or 0.5-0.8 grams per pound of your body weight per day.

Fish, eggs, lean meat, beans, and soybean foods like tofu are great sources of proteins.

Carbohydrates

When it comes to carbs, opt for complex carbohydrates. To stay healthy, try to avoid simple carbohydrates such as added sugars and refined grains which are packed with empty calories. Complex carbs are found in foods like oatmeal, whole grains, legumes (beans and lentils), sesame seeds, etc.

Fat

Dietary fat is important because it provides energy and helps with the absorption of nutrients. We have two types of fats: saturated and unsaturated. Unsaturated fats are liquid at room temperature and are considered the healthiest while saturated fats are solid at room temperature.

Choosing unsaturated fats instead of saturated ones may lower your risk of stroke and cardiovascular diseases. Some good fats that you can consume include nuts like cashew and almond or avocado. These are unsaturated fats. On the other hand, foods with saturated fats like fatty meats and shortening should be avoided.

Pre and Post Workout Nutrition

It is important to observe your pre- and post-workout nutrition. The foods you consume before and after an exercise should help you balance glucose concentration, enhance proper and faster recovery, and boost your performance. Therefore, consider a diet that is good for your body and that can efficiently supplement your workout regimen.

Pre-workout Nutrition

Before you start your exercise, you need to fuel your body with the right nutrients in their right portions depending on your training goal. This ensures that your body has enough energy to sustain your workout session and maximizes your performance.

Therefore, before your workout, consume foods that will give you enough energy up to your last exercise. The meal should contain proteins and carbs.

Each of these macronutrients plays a specific role. However, their intake ratio varies depending on your training goal and the type of exercise. For instance, if your goal is weight loss, you need to consume fewer carbs and more proteins before your workout. And if your goal is to gain muscle mass, your pre-workout diet should contain more proteins and carbs.

Let's have a look at the roles that each of these macronutrients plays when consumed before an exercise:

Carbs

Carbs fuel your muscles during an exercise. The more and harder you exercise, the more carbs you need to keep going. Carbs help control weight and provide the energy needed to run the exercises. Remember, your muscles use the glucose from carbs to fuel your body during your workout. That's why it is essential to have "good" carbs in your pre-workout diet.

Banana, oats, and whole grains are examples of "good" carbs to consume before your workout. It is recommended that you consume 0.25-0.5 grams of carbs per pound of your body weight 3-4 hours prior to your workout. But remember, this amount decreases closer to your workout. For example, you will only need 0.25 grams of carbs per pound of your body weight if you eat one hour before your workout.

Proteins

Proteins rebuild and repair our bodies. Several studies have proven that protein consumption before a workout increases muscle protein synthesis. It also enhances anabolic response, increases muscle strength and mass, and improves performance and muscle recovery.

Yogurt or protein shakes are the best ones to consume before your workout. It is recommended to consume 20 grams of protein before your exercise.

Are you wondering how soon you should eat before a workout? Ideally, you need to fuel your body with the above nutrients 1-3 hours before your workout. But, if you want to maximize the results, you are advised to consume a complete meal consisting of proteins, fats, and some carbs 2-3 hours before your workout.

If you can't get a full meal within this period, a snack also works. But if you have to eat so soon before working out, the meal should be simple to digest and smaller in portion.

Below is a list of the best foods you can consume before your workout:

- Oatmeal with low-fat milk
- Banana and mixed berries
- Whole grain bread, eggs, and brown rice
- Sandwich, lean protein, and vegetables
- Greek yogurt and fruits
- Whole-grain cereal, protein smoothie, and chicken breast

Post-workout Nutrition

As you work on your pre-workout nutrition, don't forget about your post-workout diet. To understand why it is important to eat the right foods in their right portions and proportion, you need to know how your body is affected by physical activity.

During exercise, your muscles use up their glycogen stores to fuel your body throughout the activity. This leads to partial depletion of glycogen stores in your muscles. And remember, your body needs glycogen to perform your day-to-day activities. So, after exercise, your body needs to rebuild, repair, and regrow its muscle proteins as well as replenish the depleted glycogen stores.

That's why your post-workout diet should consist of plenty of proteins with some carbs. Experts recommend eating your post-workout meals within the 45-minute window after an exercise. But the sooner you eat, the better.

Consuming a balanced diet that contains protein and a portion of carbs will replenish your glycogen stores and aid muscle growth and repair after a workout. Studies also indicate that consuming 20-40 grams of proteins after an exercise enhances speedy muscle recovery. The best protein is lean meat. Eggs are also a great option.

It is recommended to consume between 0.5-0.7 grams of carbs per pound of body weight after your workout. Some of the best carbs to consume include oatmeal, potatoes, brown rice, fruits (banana, pineapple, and berries), and chocolate. You can skip carbs after your workout and consume about 40 grams of protein if your primary goal is to lose pounds.

Some of the meals that you may consume after your workout include:

- Grilled chicken with roasted vegetables
- Low-fat yogurt with berries
- Oatmeal, wheat flakes, cereal with fruits and nuts
- Salmon with sweet potato
- Egg omelet with whole-grain toast
- Burrito with green beans
- Chicken salad with mixed greens
- Tofu with mushrooms
- Brown rice with tenderloin steak

If you consume enough macronutrients during your breakfast, lunch, and dinner, it is recommended to work out in between these meals or before your next meal. If the time between your workout and the meals is too long, consider snacks or supplements that are rich in proteins and carbs.

Supplements

When it comes to fitness, do your best to derive all your nutrients from food. Supplements are not as important as people think they are. In fact, you don't need supplements to achieve your fitness goals. However, the right ones may help speed up your results. Sound scientific studies have proved that some supplements can help you build muscles and lose fat faster, boost your performance and muscle recovery, and improve your health. Consider adding a few supplements to your workout regimen.

Creatine, beta-alanine, and citrulline have proven to help gain muscle mass and strength faster. Research has also shown that synephrine and yohimbine can help you burn more fats. On the other hand, vitamin D and fish oil improve your health and wellbeing.

In this book, I am going to focus on a few types of supplements that have been proven to be the most beneficial in achieving your health and fitness goals: fish oil, vitamin D, protein powder, fat burner, and muscle builder.

With these five types of supplements, you can improve your muscle mass and strength, lose fat, boost your immunity, improve your overall health, and more. Let's take a closer look at each of them.

1. Fish oil

Fish oil is rich in omega-3 fatty acids which are very essential for muscle building. Salmon and sardines are popular sources. Our bodies need these essential fatty acids to prevent diseases.

Research shows that on average, the diet we consume provides only a tenth of these fatty acids. That's why supplementation can be a good option. Increased levels of Omega-3 fatty acids have shown to:

- Lower depression, anxiety, and stress
- Reduce muscle and joint soreness
- Prevent excess fat gain
- Enhance fat loss
- Enhance speedy muscle gain
- Improve cognitive performance.

2. Vitamin D

Vitamin D is an essential vitamin for bone health. It helps your bones absorb calcium and can prevent osteoporosis. It also plays a big role in physiological processes like metabolism, immune system functioning, and cell growth and development. This indicates that vitamin D deficiency can lead to serious problems for your body.

We get Vitamin D from diet, sunlight, or supplementation. Vitamin D occurs naturally in a few foods like beef liver, cheese, and egg yolk, but the amount is very small. Most people get their vitamins from sunlight, but our body's ability to convert the sun's rays to vitamin D decreases as we get older. Therefore, supplementation becomes the easiest and most reliable way to add vitamin D to your body.

When it comes to other vitamin supplements, most people do not need to take them and can get the vitamins and minerals they need by eating a healthy, balanced diet.

3. Fat Burner

No pill or powder on the global market will make you healthy, stronger, and good-looking.

There is no safe "fat-burning" compound that is powerful enough to cause meaningful fat loss. Anybody claiming to sell you such a product is scamming you. Don't waste hundreds of dollars on worthless supplements peddled by steroid-fueled bodybuilders.

You shouldn't be surprised that most bodybuilding and weight loss supplements on the market are flops. Luckily, there are a few supplements that can help you accelerate your weight loss if you know how to complement it with proper dieting and exercise. Caffeine is among the few supplements that research has proven to be effective in this area.

4. Muscle Builders

Most of the popular supplements in the market that claim to aid muscle building do nothing. Fortunately, we have a few that research has proven to be effective. Creatine is among the very few you can use to accelerate muscle gain.

5. Protein Powder

You may invest in a good protein powder if you have a hard time eating enough proteins from your diet (for example, you could be allergic to most of them). There are various protein powders on the market, including vegan-friendly ones. Protein powders ensure that you are getting enough proteins to build your muscles effectively. Just add a scoop to your favorite drink and you'll be good to go! 20 grams of whey protein is beneficial when consumed before or after your workout.

Hydration

Water is essential to the human body. About 70 percent of your body composition is water. Exercise speeds up the rate at which we lose water, through sweating during and after exercise.

Therefore, considering a proper hydration strategy as part of your workout plan is important for the achievement of your fitness goals.

Staying properly hydrated is not only a requirement during exercise but it is also essential in our everyday life. "Water is life." Inadequate fluid intake leads to dehydration which can mess with your body's proper functioning. Dehydration means losing body fluids and electrolytes. Your body can't function properly without these essential important elements.

Dehydration during exercise can lead to decreased performance as it makes you feel fatigued and lazy. It also triggers muscle cramps and headaches. Besides, if you work out when you are not properly hydrated, you risk losing muscular endurance and strength.

Importance of body hydration

● It helps maximize your workout performance. Dehydration can lead to increased fatigue, muscle cramps, reduced motivation, and altered body temperatures. These make exercise feel more difficult, physically and mentally. Drinking enough water and other important fluids helps prevent dehydration thus making exercise easier to undertake.

● Water speeds up the breakdown of foods and the absorption of nutrients consumed before and after exercise, aiding faster digestion.

● Water and other fluids are great sources of important minerals and electrolytes that we lose through sweating during exercise.

- Hydration lubricates joints, enabling them to go through a full range of motion during exercise. Water also acts as a shock absorber.
- Water also helps with weight loss. Several studies have shown that drinking a glass of water before a meal decreases appetite and boosts metabolism, aiding weight loss.
- Proper hydration helps keep your skin healthy.

Ideally, you are supposed to drink 8 glasses, which equates to two liters, of water daily.

Key Takeaways

- Proper dieting doesn't mean denying yourself what you like and sticking to tasteless foods. You can get and stay in shape while eating the foods that you love.

- Different people have different nutritional needs depending on their body types, age, and fitness goals.

- As you structure a diet plan, work with what you already have.

- It is recommended to take your pre-workout meals 2-3 hours before your workout.

- Take your post-workout meals within 45 minutes after working out. The sooner the better.

• You do not need supplements if you have a good diet. Try as much as possible to get all your nutrients from a whole food diet.

• No pill or powder can make you healthy, stronger, and good-looking.

(Refer to my books "Healthy Eating for Men" or "MACRO Diet" for more information on Nutrition)

Chapter 9: Consistency is Key

"A small daily task, if it be really daily, will beat the
labors of a spasmodic Hercules."
~Anthony Trollope

Above all, be consistent. Consistency is the key to success. Consistency is key to achieving any kind of fitness goal, be it gaining muscle mass and strength, weight loss, or any other personal goal. It takes constant effort and a commitment to your training program to make the most out of your exercises.

Muscle growth usually occurs gradually with time. It is only when you stay consistent that your stamina will increase, and your exercises will be more effective and efficient. Avoid taking long breaks from your workouts.

Having a simple workout plan (which we have explored in chapter 6) is the first step in attaining consistency.

The plan for every workout is well outlined so that you will not have the burden of thinking so much about the exercises you have to perform or what you will have to do in your next workout.

A good workout plan should also focus on exercises that work out your entire body. My suggested plan in chapter 6 does just that. However, it is important to know that you may have the most effective and perfect workout plan in place, but if you can't be consistent and adhere to it, it is not going to benefit you in any way.

When you consistently perform intense exercises, your muscles get injured from the training. This disrupts your muscle cell organelles, which in turn activates the satellite cells. The satellite cells then get stimulated by your body's hormones, which increase the size of your muscle fibers.

We all desire a strong, healthy, and good-looking body. But you have to understand that you need to embrace consistency to achieve your goals. To be consistent with your workout, you need to make it a habit. The more frequently you perform the exercises, the more natural it becomes.

In the beginning, things may seem tough. You may even be tempted to quit. Don't. Just remember you need consistency to unlock success in your training goals and the rest will fall in place. Once your body adapts, that's all. In fact, you will never want to miss your workout.

Tips for Staying Consistent

- **Plan for obstacles.** Think about all the possible events that would force you to take longer breaks from working out and plan for them. Be proactive. We all encounter stumbling blocks in our daily life. Having a plan on how to address these obstacles prepares you physically and psychologically to move forward.

- **Use reminders.** When you've just started on a new thing that is not part of your daily grind, it is very easy to forget about them. You may forget that you need to work out on a particular day. Sometimes you may even forget that you have a workout program that you're following. To avoid forgetting to exercise, set reminders on your phone, calendar, watch, or even smart assistants. You can also print your workout program and stick it close to your mirror, refrigerator, or office desk.

- **Avoid negative thoughts.** Every success starts with your mind. What you think is what you are. Most of us allow our minds to sabotage our plans and goals. If you understand the saying "we are our worst enemies," then you will understand what I am talking about. If your mindset is, "I can't...", "I am not..." and predominantly negative, you are less likely to exercise consistently.

- **Be committed.** Commitment means doing something even if you don't feel like doing it, you don't like it, or when it is inconvenient. If you want to achieve consistency in your workout, you have to stay committed to exercising for at least 30 days. Whether you exercise, once, twice, or three times a week, doing it for a month will help you stick with the exercise. Are you wondering why a month? Research has proven that it takes 24 days of doing something repeatedly to make it a habit.

• **Set your goal.** Concentrate more on setting short-term goals. Some long-term goals may be unrealistic and may seem unachievable. Write your goal down and check to ensure it is SMART (Specific – Measurable – Achievable – Relevant – Time-limited). Connect it to something significant in your life so it takes root deep within you. Go the extra mile and highlight the reasons for the goal and the expected benefits of achieving the goal. For example, instead of having a goal like exercising frequently, plan to exercise 2-3 days a week for 30 minutes for the next 18 weeks because it is going to help you gain more muscle mass and energy, take care of yourself, and play with your children.

• **Have a good workout routine.** Starting a fitness journey without a workout routine is one of the easiest ways to fail. You've probably heard that "What gets scheduled, gets done." It is easier to say that you will exercise than it is to put it into action. It is more real when you schedule your workout on your calendar or planner. It also makes you more accountable, stay on track, and make exercise a priority.

• **Start small and progress gradually.** Do not rush into lifting heavier loads and performing more sets/reps. Take it slow. Most people who quit exercising almost always start at a pace that they can't maintain for long. Start small and as you get stronger, gradually increase the intensity of your workout, sets/reps, and weights.

- **Be patient.** You cannot build muscles overnight. Most people think they'll see results right away. Such expectations are unrealistic. You need to be patient with yourself if you notice that you're not sticking to your workout routine 100 percent. You need to understand that establishing a new habit can take time. Just trust the process and be patient.

- **Seek accountability.** People are more likely to strictly follow their workout routine when they're observed by others. To be fully committed to implementing changes, find an accountability buddy. This can be your spouse, friend, or even a family member. Nobody likes to disappoint their workout partner or someone they love. While choosing an accountability buddy, select someone who has a similar workout program.

- **Keep track of your progress.** Measure your progress weekly to find out what you've achieved. Note down any progress you make. Seeing what you have achieved will motivate you to exercise more and improve on where you feel you're not doing well.

- **Make exercise enjoyable.** Find different ways to make your workout fun. You may connect it with something pleasurable like a game, take it outdoors and do it with friends, or reward yourself to reinforce your regular effort.

You need to make exercise part of your life to achieve a healthier, stronger, fitter, and leaner body. The tips above will help you stay consistent with your workout and experience long-lasting change.

Workout Stagnation

There are times when our bodies reach a stagnation point. Workout stagnation simply means that you strictly follow your workout routine, but you can't see any change. Stagnation usually occurs when your muscles get adapted to a defined workout plan and the same stimuli. As a result, your workout performance decreases, your muscles stop growing, and your body fails to register any progress in muscle gain.

Workout stagnation is common and normal. When you reach a stagnation point, you need to change your workout strategy and approach. Here is what you should do:

- **Up your sets /reps.** If you've been doing 3 sets of 6 reps, increase that to 4 sets or 10 reps using lighter weights. It is advisable to change your reps/sets as you progress while your body adapts.

- **Warm up before you start exercising.** Stimulate your muscles by performing some warmup exercises like jogging in place before you begin your workout.

- **Adjust your workout routine.** Redefine and modify your current workout plan using alternative exercises from chapter 4. All we are trying to do here is to exercise our muscles through different angles. This gives your body new stimuli for muscle growth.

- **Create a diet plan that backs up your workout.** Have a diet plan in place that helps supply your body with the necessary energy and nutrients before and after your workout.

- **Lower your repetition speed.** This enables your muscles to experience more time under tension, enabling them to go through a full range of motion.

- **Try completing your exercises in the less expected time.** Performing more exercises in less time helps expose your muscles to new stimuli allowing them room to grow.

- **Create a balance between volume and intensity.** Never neglect your body. If your workout intensity is high, reduce the number of sessions you do in a week, and if the intensity is low, increase the sessions.

When you subject your muscles to certain exercise intensity, your body responds by forming new muscles to cope with the situation at hand. But note that the stress on these forces is continuous and repeated, which means your body has to keep forming new muscles. This means that you will need to be consistent with your workout to help your muscles become stronger to cope with the stress.

It is so gratifying when you are consistent. On the other hand, it is so frustrating when you fail to accomplish it since you fail to achieve your goal.

Remember, consistency is a skill you learn through patience. Just endure all the challenges that come along as you work out and you will achieve consistency.

Key Takeaways

- Consistency is your strongest weapon in the battle to achieve your strength training goals. Stay consistent with your workout plan, nutrition, and recovery.

Chapter 10: FAQs

"If you think lifting is dangerous, try being weak. Being weak is dangerous."
~ Bret Contreras

Q1: I haven't exercised for all my years, isn't it too late to start now?

It is never too late. Even if you've never exercised, you can start now and you will reap the same benefits that other people who strength train while younger do. Experts assure us that seniors who have had a sedentary lifestyle can start a regular workout regimen at any age.

I am not encouraging you to wait until you're 80 to begin to exercise. Remember, if you wait that long, you're causing harm to yourself. All your muscles will be gone. Strength training will help preserve your muscles and bone health. Research also shows that you can still lower the risks of age-related health problems if you begin your exercise regimen when you're older.

Q2: I am not overweight. Do I really need to work out?

You might not be overweight, but you might be weak or have other bone-related health issues. Being thin doesn't equate a healthy and fit body. What I mean is that to maintain good health and reduce health risks, you need to exercise regularly, even if your doctor confirms that your weight is healthy. A sedentary lifestyle increases the risk of developing age-related health problems. So, regular exercise is key, whether you are overweight or not.

Q3: I have several medical problems. Is it safe to exercise?

It is advisable to consult your doctor before you start any workout program. Explain your condition and ask about any specific precautions you need to take and the exercises that are safe for you.

Research shows that regular exercise can help minimize the risk of chronic illnesses and speed up the recovery process of serious diseases like heart attack, stroke, joint-replacement surgery, and many more. That's why you may find many doctors recommending exercise even after a serious injury or illness.

Exercise also helps fight osteoporosis, keeps your body limber, and joints stabilized, preventing injuries. So, the simple answer to this question is: Exercise is safe and beneficial even if you have medical conditions; in fact, it will help you manage those conditions.

Q4: Do I really need exercise at this age?

You are never too old. There is no age limit to becoming fit. You can strength train at any age and still reap the many benefits that come with it. In fact, staying physically inactive is more dangerous and has been proven to hasten the aging process. People who exercise are twice less likely to contract chronic illnesses than those who don't exercise.

You need more regular exercise now than when you were younger. Your metabolism is slower, you lose muscle mass each passing year and fat now tends to accumulate so easily. Your bones are delicate and more susceptible to fracture. This means that you must do something.

Q5. How long does it take to lose muscle when you stop training?

Once you get started on your strength training routine, you might worry about losing your hard-earned muscle mass and strength if you take a break. Taking a few days off from exercising isn't bad for you, in fact, it helps you achieve your fitness goals as it gives your muscles time to recover. However, the problem is when we take too long breaks.

If you take too long without training, some research suggests that you can start to lose muscle within one week of inactivity - as much as two pounds if you are fully immobilized. Another study suggests that your muscle size can decrease by about 11% after ten days without exercise, even when you aren't bedridden.

Before you panic and regret every vacation or week off you've taken, it is important to understand that true muscle atrophy typically takes place during times of injury or when you completely stop using your muscles for an extended period. You can take about three weeks off without seeing a noticeable drop in your muscle strength.

However, how quickly you lose muscles mass when you stop training is determined by different factors, including:

• **How long and often you've been training.** The time you've been training determines the muscles you have. If you've been consistent with weightlifting for a longer period, it means you have more muscles. This puts you in a better position even if you need to pause your routine.

• **Your diet.** We need adequate protein to build and maintain muscle mass. People with protein deficiencies lack adequate amino acids to keep up with the constant breakdown and rebuilding of body cells that goes on every day. Eventually, your body pulls the amino acids stored in your muscles and uses them to keep other cells and tissues functioning. This results in muscle loss. So, it is very important to ensure that you are getting enough proteins even if you're not training.

• **Age.** Many age-related changes make it harder to build and maintain muscle mass. The change in our nervous system coordination is one of them. As we get older, we tend to lose motor neurons. Motor neurons enhance muscle contractions by transmitting impulses from the spinal cord to the muscles. Therefore, if you lose them, recruiting muscle fibers becomes difficult. So, strength training helps reverse these changes and many other age-related changes. However, if you stop training, the benefits disappear gradually.

• **Sex**. Since males have natural testosterone, which is anabolic to muscle tissue development and maintenance, they have a slight advantage compared to females when it comes to muscle loss.

Q6. How do I select the right weight—Kettlebell?

You are allowed to test whether you can bear the weight of the kettlebell you want to use in your workout or not. To select a good weight, try to do several reps of kettlebell military press in the shop. The weight you will manage is the right one. Although you will need the smallest weight for this exercise, this weight will be suitable for the rest of the exercises too. Remember, it is better to start small and master the moves instead of injuring yourself.

Q7. Can Testosterone Replacement Therapy (TRT) improve my workout results?

Yes. In fact, most of the men I have met with well-built bodies confess that TRT is their secret. When you reach 30, your testosterone hormone levels decline by about 1% every year, and this increases gradually with age (Mayo Clinic, 2020). So, if you realize that you have abnormally low testosterone, you may need to boost it to gain the most out of your weightlifting exercises.

However, I don't recommend TRT. I prefer boosting your testosterone levels naturally. We all know that anything done naturally has little to no side effects. Research shows that TRT may lead to lower sperm count, increased risk of a blood clot and heart attack, stimulation of noncancerous prostate growth, enlarged breasts, testicle shrinkage, etc. If you are ready for all these, then you can opt for TRT.

One of the best ways to maintain or increase your testosterone levels is by consuming vitamins and supplements like zinc, vitamin B and D. Other ways include getting enough sleep (7-10 hours), proper diet, and exercise.

Bonus Chapter: Your Fitness, Your Way: Varied Workout Plans to Suit Every Lifestyle

I understand that no two fitness journeys are identical, and that's why I've compiled a collection of workout plans that offer something for everyone.

From bodyweight enthusiasts to gym aficionados, from those who prefer minimal equipment to those with access to a full range of tools, this chapter ensures that you find a fitness path that resonates with your unique needs. My mission is to empower you to curate your fitness journey, embracing a plan that fits seamlessly into your lifestyle, schedule, and objectives.

There are many ways of programming workouts, but one strategy has been popular for decades now. In fact, just about every time-proven strength and muscle-building program fits this basic mold, and that's not likely to change. It is called "push pull legs" or PPL routine. The primary reasons push pull legs routines have stood the test of time are they train all major muscle groups, allow plenty of time for recovery, and can be tailored to fit different training goals, schedules, and histories. They're easy to understand, too. A push pull legs routine separates your major muscle groups into three different workouts: push workout (for chest, shoulders, and triceps), pull workout (for back and biceps), and legs workout.

This program can be undertaken anywhere from two to six times per week, depending on how much you're willing to take, your physique goals, and how much time you have for working out.

The first thing to decide is how many days per week that you want to train. Athletes who want to maximize muscle and strength gains usually train five to six days per week.

But that doesn't suit everyone.

If you're short on time, don't despair – you can still do great with two to three workouts per week.

Another major benefit of push pull legs is it can be easily customized to fit your needs and circumstances.

With just three basic workouts to choose from, it's easy to grasp and add, subtract, or shift around workouts each week as needed.

A three-day routine is basic PPL program, and it's my personal favorite setup. More training is best for maximizing gains, but this three-day split is a time-proven program for getting lean and strong.

For example, the most basic **3-day setup** looks like this:

Monday: **PUSH**

Tuesday: Rest

Wednesday: **PULL**

Thursday: Rest

Friday: **LEGS**

Saturday: Rest

Sunday: Rest

More would be better if you're trying to gain muscle and strength as quickly as possible, but when circumstances won't allow for more gym time, a solid two-day routine can help you at least maintain what you've got. As I mentioned earlier, you can do well training just twice per week. If you want to train just **two days per week**, you could do something like this:

Monday: Rest

Tuesday: **PUSH & LEGS**

Wednesday: Rest

Thursday: Rest

Friday: **PULL**

Saturday: Rest

Sunday: Rest

Or, if you want to push yourself to your limits, you could do something like this **six-day setup**:

Monday: **PUSH**

Tuesday: **PULL**

Wednesday: **LEGS**

Thursday: **PUSH**

Friday: **PULL**

Saturday: **LEGS**

Sunday: Rest

Five-day split* allows you also to push the limits in terms of volume and intensity while also allowing a couple days for recovery:

Monday: **PUSH**

Tuesday: **PULL**

Wednesday: **LEGS**

Thursday: Rest

Friday: **PUSH**

Saturday: **PULL**

Sunday: Rest

And a **four-day split*** allows three days per week for recovery:

Monday: **PUSH**

Tuesday: **PULL**

Wednesday: Rest

Thursday: **LEGS**

Friday: **PUSH**

Saturday: Rest

Sunday: Rest

In these four- and five-day workout routines you start every new week with a different workout (with the one that goes next in order to stick to training sequence: push, pull, legs, push, pull, legs, etc.)

I'm going to provide two alternative four-day routines: one for people that want to focus more on their upper bodies (most often – men), and one for focusing more on the lower body (most often – women). Compared to basic three-day PPL workout routine, the major benefit of adding a fourth day is you get to work more on whichever major muscles groups you need, or want, to focus most on:

Four-day split with upper body focus:

Monday: **PUSH**

Tuesday: **PULL**

Wednesday: Rest

Thursday: **LEGS**

Friday: **PUSH**

Saturday: Rest

Sunday: Rest

Four-day split with lower body focus:

Monday: **LEGS**

Tuesday: **PUSH**

Wednesday: Rest

Thursday: **PULL**

Friday: **LEGS**

Saturday: Rest

Sunday: Rest

Once you've decided how many days you're going to train each week, the next step is selecting a specific workout plan. There are many ways of programming push pull legs, but I'm going to keep it simple and give you a few templates of my favorites. Just pick the one that best suits your fitness level, favorite equipment, and personal preferences.

I'm sure you will find a plan that you can easily follow to add some weight training to your weekly routine.

You will discover bodyweight workouts that leverage your own strength, kettlebell routines that add dynamism to your training, dumbbell exercises that sculpt and tone, and resistance band workouts that pack a punch in minimal space or when on the move. For those on the move or preferring the comfort of their home, I've curated workouts tailored to these preferences. And if you're drawn to the structured environment of a gym, we've got you covered with barbell workouts and gym equipment-based routines that offer an array of possibilities.

Not everyone who wants to get fitter and stronger can (or wants) go to a gym. And if this is the case for you, a bodyweight workout routine is a great option.

If you're new to exercise, I recommend starting with the bodyweight workout for beginners.

BODYWEIGHT WORKOUT FOR BEGINNERS:
3-DAY SPLIT

DAY 1: PUSH	
Push-Up	3 sets of 10-20 reps
Knee Push-Up	3 sets of 10-20 reps
Triceps "Bench" Dip	3 sets of 10-20 reps
DAY 2: PULL	
Negative Chin-Up	3 sets of 10-20 reps
Bodyweight Row	3 sets of 10-20 reps
Isometric Chin-Up	3 sets of 10-20 reps
DAY 3: LEGS	
Bodyweight Squat	3 sets of 10-20 reps
Bodyweight Glute Bridge	3 sets of 10-20 reps
Bodyweight Calf Raise	3 sets of 10-20 reps

If you've got experience with bodyweight training or weightlifting and you're looking for a challenging bodyweight workout routine, then the advanced workout routine will likely suit you best.

ADVANCED BODYWEIGHT WORKOUT: 3-DAY SPLIT

DAY 1: PUSH	
Feet Elevated Push-Up	3 sets of 10-20 reps
Diamond Push-Up	3 sets of 10-20 reps
Push-Up	3 sets of 10-20 reps
DAY 2: PULL	
Pull-Up	3 sets of 10-20 reps
Bodyweight Row	3 sets of 10-20 reps
Chin-Up	3 sets of 10-20 reps
DAY 3: LEGS	
Bodyweight Bulgarian Split Squat	3 sets of 10-20 reps
Bodyweight Squat	3 sets of 10-20 reps
Bodyweight Glute Bridge	3 sets of 10-20 reps

There are a lot of people who only do bodyweight exercises and are in a great shape.

However, if you are serious about shaping up and building body strength, then it is worthwhile to invest in at least one or two pieces of equipment to get the most out of your exercise routine.

A kettlebell, a dumbbell, a barbell, or a resistance band is a great choice!

In next pages you will find workouts that you can do with these tools.

1 KETTLEBELL (OR 1 DUMBELL) WORKOUT: 3-DAY SPLIT

DAY 1: PUSH	
Push-Up	3 sets of 10-20 reps
Right arm Military Press	3 sets of 6-10 reps
Left Arm Military Press	3 sets of 6-10 reps
DAY 2: PULL	
Right Arm Kettlebell Row	3 sets of 6-10 reps
Left Arm Kettlebell Row	3 sets of 6-10 reps
Kettlebell Swing	3 sets of 6-10 reps
DAY 3: LEGS & CORE	
Kettlebell Goblet Squat	3 sets of 6-10 reps
Leg Raise or Crunch	3 sets of 10-20 reps

1 KETTLEBELL (OR 1 DUMBELL) WORKOUT: 2-DAY SPLIT

DAY 1: PUSH & LEGS	
Push-Up	3 sets of 10-20 reps
Kettlebell Goblet Squats	3 sets of 6-10 reps
Right Arm Military Press	3 sets of 6-10 reps
Left Arm Military Press	3 sets of 6-10 reps
DAY 2: RULL & CORE	
Right Arm Kettlebell Row	3 sets of 6-10 reps
Left Arm Kettlebell Row	3 sets of 6-10 reps
Kettlebell Swings	3 sets of 6-10 reps
Leg Raise or Crunch	3 sets of 10-20 reps

2 DUMBELLS (OR 2 KETTLEBELLS) WORKOUT: 3-DAY SPLIT

DAY 1: PUSH	
Dumbbell Chest Press	3 sets of 6-10 reps
Dumbbell Shoulder Press	3 sets of 6-10 reps
DAY 2: PULL	
Bent-Over Dumbbell Row	3 sets of 6-10 reps
Dumbbell Deadlift	3 sets of 6-10 reps
DAY 3: LEGS & CORE	
Dumbbell Squat	3 sets of 6-10 reps
Leg Raise or Crunch	3 sets of 10-20 reps

2 DUMBELLS (OR 2 KETTLEBELLS) WORKOUT: 2-DAY SPLIT

DAY 1: PUSH & LEGS	
Dumbbell Chest Press	3 sets of 6-10 reps
Dumbbell Shoulder Press	3 sets of 6-10 reps
Dumbbell Squat	3 sets of 6-10 reps
DAY 2: PULL & CORE	
Bent-Over Dumbbell Row	3 sets of 6-10 reps
Dumbbell Deadlift	3 sets of 6-10 reps
Leg Raise or Crunch	3 sets of 10-20 reps

RESISTANCE BAND WORKOUT: 3-DAY SPLIT

DAY 1: PUSH	
Push-Up with Resistance	3 sets of 6-10 reps
Lateral Raise	3 sets of 6-10 reps
Triceps Extension	3 sets of 6-10 reps
DAY 2: PULL	
Deadlift	3 sets of 6-10 reps
Row	3 sets of 6-10 reps
Bicep Curl	3 sets of 6-10 reps
DAY 3: LEGS & CORE	
Squat with Resistance	3 sets of 6-10 reps
Leg Raise or Crunch	3 sets of 10-20 reps

RESISTANCE BAND WORKOUT: 2-DAY SPLIT

DAY 1: PUSH & LEGS	
Push-Up with Resistance	3 sets of 6-10 reps
Lateral Raise	3 sets of 6-10 reps
Triceps Extension	3 sets of 6-10 reps
Squat with Resistance	3 sets of 6-10 reps
DAY 2: PULL & CORE	
Deadlift	3 sets of 6-10 reps
Row	3 sets of 6-10 reps
Bicep Curl	3 sets of 6-10 reps
Leg Raise or Crunch	3 sets of 10-20 reps

BARBELL WORKOUT: 3-DAY SPLIT

DAY 1: PUSH	
Incline Barbell Bench Press	3 sets of 6-10 reps
Seated Barbell Shoulder Press	3 sets of 6-10 reps
Lying Triceps Extension	3 sets of 6-10 reps
Dumbbell Side Lateral Raise	3 sets of 6-10 reps
DAY 2: PULL & CORE	
Deadlift	3 sets of 6-10 reps
Pull-Up	3 sets of 6-10 reps
Barbell Bent-Over Row	3 sets of 6-10 reps
Leg Raise or Crunch	3 sets of 10-20 reps
DAY 3: LEGS	
Barbell Squat	3 sets of 6-10 reps
Romanian Deadlift	3 sets of 6-10 reps
Dumbbell Lunge	3 sets of 6-10 reps
Standing Barbell Calf Raise	3 sets of 6-10 reps

BARBELL WORKOUT: 2-DAY SPLIT

DAY 1: PUSH & LEGS	
Incline Barbell Bench Press	3 sets of 6-10 reps
Barbell Squat	3 sets of 6-10 reps
Seated Barbell Shoulder Press	3 sets of 6-10 reps
Parallel Bars Triceps Dips	3 sets of 6-10 reps
Leg Raise	3 sets of 10-20 reps
DAY 2: PUSH & CORE	
Deadlift	3 sets of 6-10 reps
Pull Up	3 sets of 6-10 reps
Barbell Bent-Over Row	3 sets of 6-10 reps
Barbell Bicep Curl	3 sets of 6-10 reps
Crunch	3 sets of 10-20 reps

If you're not sure how to perform some of the exercises – don't worry. To make things simple, I've linked the workouts from this book to videos that show proper form of each exercise in a downloadable PDF.

To get instant access to it, go to **"Free Bonus Material"**.

Free Bonus Material

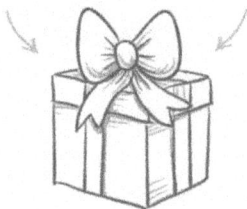

Thank you for reading *Strength Training over 40*.

I hope you find it insightful, inspiring, and practical, and I hope it helps you build that strong and healthy body you really desire.

To help you get the best results as fast as possible, I've put together additional free resources:

1. Strength Training Workout Routines with Links to Form Demonstration Videos for Exercises
2. Macro Friendly Grocery List to never run out of ideas about what to eat
3. 6-Step Quick Start Guide to finally take your fitness under control
4. Daily Checklist to stay on track with your fitness goals
5. Example Meal Plan to supercharge your fat loss
6. Comprehensive Workout LogSheet for keeping track of your workouts
7. Top Tips for Seniors to enjoy your life and avoid health problems as you age

To get your bonuses go to link:

bit.ly/3P4LC8n

or scan QR code with your camera

Conclusion

"All progress takes place outside the comfort zone."
~ Michael John Bobak

The innumerable benefits of strength training can never be overemphasized. No matter your age, it is never too late.

With strength training, you can build muscle mass, manage chronic illnesses, improve bone strength and health, and more. If you want to stay healthy, strong and in good shape, this book has got you covered.

Strength training is the way to go if you want to achieve these three things—a strong, healthy, and fit body. You might find it intimidating to make this kind of commitment if you're new to strength training because it forces you out of your warm comfort zone, but that is the only choice that you have if you want to achieve this precious goal. Just approach it with the right mindset and you will succeed!

Key Takeaways

• You need to find the right motivation. Find your fitness whys. By doing so, you will be able to do whatever it takes to achieve them. You may find creating time for training a herculean task, but if you plan well, you will find yourself with an abundance of it.

• As you start your training, go slowly and steadily. Set smart goals and stick to working hard towards achieving them. Remember, you are more likely to fail if you don't have a purpose or destination in mind. Visualize one. And as you begin your training, be patient. Good things take time, so does achieving a strong, healthy, and fit body. It takes years for a bottle of fine wine to mature. So, exercise patience!

• You don't need a lot of equipment to exercise. Strength training does not require fancy or expensive weightlifting equipment or gym-style machines. However, it is a wise idea to invest in a few pieces of equipment.

• You don't need to spend a lot of money on expensive equipment. With just one kettlebell, you have everything you need to make incredible gains from your training program without draining your pocket. You will find it is worth your investment and you will never regret it. Although you can still achieve your strength training goal without any equipment (using your body weight), I believe that using free weights, especially a kettlebell, is the most effective option.

• Have a workout plan. Anyone who fails to plan, plans to fail. I have designed a workout plan for YOU. To get the full benefits of strength training, make sure you try this plan for at least four weeks. It will help you stay on course and train effectively. Be consistent, and remember to progressively overload your muscles with higher weights, reps, or sets.

• Follow a proper diet plan. Never underestimate the power of nutrition and its impacts on the achievement of your fitness goals. Remember, your diet will either make or break your strength training goals. Be careful with what you consume. This doesn't mean denying yourself your favorite foods and sticking to tasteless foods. You can keep fit while consuming the foods that you love.

• There are beneficial nutrients your body needs that you must prioritize, and if you can't have enough from the food you consume, take supplements. However, I encourage people to do their best to get all their nutrients from whole foods, not supplementation.

• Stay away from processed foods. Avoid sugary and processed foods because they will worsen your health.

- Consume between 1.2-1.7 grams of protein per kilogram of your body weight goal or 0.5-0.8 grams per pound of your goal body weight per day.

- Consume 20-40 grams of proteins before and after your workout.

- Performing your exercises in supersets is the best way to save time while getting the most out of your workout.

- You need to perform three sets of 6-12 reps to reap the benefits of both muscle and strength building.

- You also need to train 1-3 days per week with rest days in between.

- As you exercise, **do it safely**. Remember, the goal here is to sustain fitness, muscle mass, strength, and good health, not sustaining injuries. Ensure you exercise properly. Don't push too hard too soon. Start small and work your way up. Use proper form while executing the moves. Your safety is very important. Don't overuse your muscles. Allow them enough time to recover.

- Be consistent. Remember consistency is your strongest weapon in achieving your desired body.

- **Lastly, stay properly hydrated.** Drink enough water before, during, and after exercise to prevent dehydration. Ideally, drink two liters of water daily.

Strength training combined with proper nutrition, recovery, and hydration is guaranteed to get you to your fitness goals. Just be consistent and ensure you carry out your workouts safely.

Now that you have all it takes to build that strong, fit, and healthy body, go out and hunt for it. You need to put more effort into applying what you've learned in this book, otherwise, the information herein will be powerless to change your physique and your life. The most important thing in anybody's life is to have fun and be happy doing the things that they love. Hopefully, strength training can be one of those things just like it is for me.

CAN I ASK YOU FOR A FAVOR?

Thank you for reading this book.

I have a small favor to ask.

If you enjoyed this book and have benefitted from it in any way, please take a few moments to post a review on Amazon.

With this small gesture, you are helping me reach more people who are going to benefit from this book.

I check all my reviews and love to get your feedback.

That's the real pay for my work – knowing that I'm helping people.

To leave a quick review go to link:

amazon.com/dp/B09M731H1C

Or scan QR code with your camera:

At **BODY YOU DESERVE Publishing**, we strongly believe that there are a thousand ways to improve your life and health. However, there is no single recipe suitable for everyone how to do that.

We think that the best way to receive your goals is the one you can stick to, and our writers do their best to provide simple, easy to follow, step by step, and realistic instructions.

To discover our best books, go to link:

https://amzn.to/40B5KmZ

Or scan QR code with your camera:

References

Barhum, L. (2018, July 18). *How do you boost testosterone naturally?* MEDICALNEWSTODAY. https://www.medicalnewstoday.com/articles/322508#natural-ways-to-maintain-testosterone

Beabout, L. (2020, August 27). *Knee Push-Ups 101: Lighten Your Load and Still Feel the Burn*. Greatist. https://greatist.com/fitness/knee-pushup#how-to

Bedosky, L. (2020, November 11). *How Long Does It Take to Lose Muscle? | Fitness | MyFitnessPal*. MyFitnessPal Blog. https://blog.myfitnesspal.com/how-long-does-it-take-to-lose-muscle/

Briley, J. (2020, June 9). *You're never too old to regain that lost muscle. And you can do it at home*. Washington Post. Retrieved November 15, 2021, from https://www.washingtonpost.com/lifestyle/wellness/youre-never-too-old-to-regain-that-lost-muscle-and-you-can-do-it-at-home/2020/06/05/b221ccc4-a5d1-11ea-bb20-ebf0921f3bbd_story.html

Collins, A. (2020). *Strength Training Over 40: A 6-Week Program to Build Muscle and Agility*. Rockridge Press.

Collins, S. (2012, May 14). *The Truth About Stretching*. WebMD. https://www.webmd.com/fitness-exercise/features/how-to-stretch#1

Dobbins, C. (2018). *The Simple Six: The Easy Way to Get in Shape and Stay in Shape for the Rest of your Life*. Independently published.

Dunkin, M. A. (2009, October 1). *Sarcopenia With Aging*. WebMD. Retrieved November 15, 2021, from https://www.webmd.com/healthy-aging/guide/sarcopenia-with-aging

Emma, F. (2020). *Fitness Over 40: Build More Muscle, Strength & Agility While Supercharging Your Health As A 40, 50 Or 60+ Year Old Using These Strength Training Exercises & Nutrition Guides*. Independently published.

Fetters, A. K. (2019, October 16). *8 Benefits of Doing Free Weights Exercises*. Shape. https://www.shape.com/fitness/tips/benefits-of-free-weights-vs-machine

Fuel during and after exercise. (n.d.). Mayo Clinic Health System. https://www.mayoclinichealthsystem.org/hometown-health/speaking-of-health/monday-run-day-11-fuel-during-and-after-exercise

Hip Raises / Butt Lift / Bridges – WorkoutLabs Exercise Guide. (n.d.). WorkoutLabs. https://workoutlabs.com/exercise-guide/hip-raises/

Kamb, S. (2021a, July 18). *How Many Sets and Reps Should I Do? (Building a Workout)*. Nerd Fitness. https://www.nerdfitness.com/blog/the-correct-number-of-reps-per-set-in-the-gym/

Kamb, S. (2021b, July 18). *How Many Sets and Reps Should I Do? (Building a Workout)*. Nerd Fitness. https://www.nerdfitness.com/blog/the-correct-number-of-reps-per-set-in-the-gym/

Kawamoto, J. (2019, June 7). *5 Methods to Make Progress With Your Workouts*. Muscle & Fitness. https://www.muscleandfitness.com/workouts/workout-tips/5-methods-progress-your-workouts/

Know When to Take Your Strength Training to the Next Level. (2021, May 27). Verywell Fit. https://www.verywellfit.com/progression-definition-3120367

Lisa, S. (2021). *Fitness Over 40: A Six-Week Exercise Plan to Build Endurance, Strength, & Flexibility*. Rockridge Press.

MacPherson, R. (2021, June 9). *How often should you strength train to build muscle and avoid injury*.

Insider. https://www.insider.com/how-often-should-you-strength-train

Magnante, M. (2021, September 11). *Kettlebell Arnold Press Exercise Guide and Videos*. Fitness Volt. https://fitnessvolt.com/kettlebell-arnold-press/

Martinez, M. (2020, November 11). *Kettlebell Goblet Squat: How To Do It & Get Ripped*. Onnit Academy. https://www.onnit.com/academy/kettlebell-goblet-squat/

Matthews, M. (2021). *Bigger Leaner Stronger: The Simple Science of Building the Ultimate Male Body*. Waterbury Publications, Inc.

McDermott, N. (2014, November 10). *How to Do the Perfect Plank*. Greatist. https://greatist.com/fitness/perfect-plank#fix-common-mistakes

Publishing, W. A., & Carney, W. D. (2020). *Mature Muscle: Ultimate Training Manual to Build Muscle over 40*. Wisdom Authority Publishing.

Pugle, M. (2019, March 15). *Getting Into Shape After Age 40: The Best Ways to Do It*. Healthline. https://www.healthline.com/health-news/how-to-finally-get-in-shape-after-40

Reyes, A. M. (2021). *Strength Over 40: Strength Training for the Better Half of Your Life, 67 Exercises to Improve Flexibility, Mobility and Increase Strength (Women's Edition)*. Independently published.

Romine, S. (2020, June 23). *Bored with Push-Ups? Try the Pike Push-Up*. Greatist. https://greatist.com/health/pike-pushups#how-to-do-it

Salter, M. P. S., & Salter, M. P. S. (2020, August 17). *Time Your Carbs Perfectly To Crush Your Goals*. Bodybuilding.Com. https://www.bodybuilding.com/fun/time-your-carbs-perfectly-to-crush-your-goals

Semeco, M. A. S. (2021, April 12). *Post-Workout Nutrition: What to Eat After a Workout*. Healthline. https://www.healthline.com/nutrition/eat-after-workout

Simic, L. (2013, March 1). *Does preexercise static stretching inhibit maximal muscular performance? A meta analytical review*. Wiley Online Library. https://onlinelibrary.wiley.com/doi/10.1111/j.1600-0838.2012.01444.x

Smith, K. (2020, September 29). *Burn 400 Calories in 20 Minutes With Kettlebells*. Kathy Smith. https://www.kathysmith.com/burn-400-calories-in-20-minutes-with-kettlebells/

Smith, M. (2020). *Healthy Eating for Men: Get Back in Shape, Prevent Health problems, Lose Weight and Stay Fit at Any Age (Health & Wellness)*. Independently published.

Stevens, E. (2017, June 2). *5 Ways to Find Your Fitness "Why."* Muscle and Performance. https://www.muscleandperformance.com/training/5-ways-to-find-your-fitness-why/

Sullivan, J. C., & Sullivan, J. C. (2021, November 2). *This Simple Pushup Tweak Makes Your Shoulders Burn Like Crazy*. Women's Health. https://www.womenshealthmag.com/fitness/a34975918/decline-push-up/

SWEAT. (2019, September 26). *One-Arm Kettlebell Row*. https://www.sweat.com/blogs/exercises/one-arm-kettlebell-row

T. (2015, February 5). *HIIT Exercise: How To Do Feet Elevated Pike Push Ups | HIIT Academy | HIIT Workouts | HIIT Workouts For Men | HIIT Workouts For Women | HIIT Training*. HIITACADEMY. https://hiitacademy.com/hiit-exercise-how-to-do-feet-elevated-pike-push-ups/

Testosterone therapy: Potential benefits and risks as you age. (2020, April 4). Mayo Clinic.

http://mayoclinic.org/healthy-lifestyle/sexual-health/in-depth/testosterone-therapy/art-20045728?reDate=17112021

Thompson, B. (2018). *Strength Training After 40: A Practical Guide to Building and Maintaining a Healthier, Leaner, and Stronger Body*. Baz Thompson.

Week, T. O. T., & Week, T. O. T. (2021, March 5). *What Is The Optimal Time Between Sets For Muscle Growth?* Bodybuilding.Com. https://www.bodybuilding.com/content/what-is-the-optimal-time-between-sets-for-muscle-growth.html

Westcott, W., & Baechle, T. R. (2015). *Strength Training Past 50* (Third ed.). Human Kinetics.

What is Supersetting and Why You Should Try It. (n.d.). In-Shape. https://www.inshape.com/member-buzz/what-is-supersetting-and-why-you-should-try-it/

Image Credit: Gym Visual

www.ingramcontent.com/pod-product-compliance
Ingram Content Group UK Ltd.
Pitfield, Milton Keynes, MK11 3LW, UK
UKHW031430020125
3922UKWH00046B/1011

9 798773 536086